100 CASES
in Paediatrics

100 CASES
in Paediatrics

J. E. Raine MD FRCPCH DCH
Consultant Paediatrician, Whittington Hospital, London;
Honorary Senior Lecturer, University College, London, UK

A. J. Cunnington BMBCh MA MRCPCH DTM&H
Specialist Registrar in Paediatrics, London Deanery;
Clinical Research Fellow, Immunology Unit,
London School of Hygiene and Tropical Medicine, London, UK

J. M. Walker BA FRCP FRCPCH
Consultant Paediatrician, Portsmouth Hospitals NHS Trust,
Portsmouth, UK

Volume Editor:
J. E. Raine

100 Cases Series Editor:
P. John Rees M FRCP
Dean of Medical Undergraduate Education, King's College London
School of Medicine at Guy's, King's and St Thomas' Hospitals, London, UK

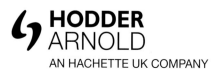
HODDER
ARNOLD
AN HACHETTE UK COMPANY

First published in Great Britain in 2009 by
Hodder Arnold, an imprint of Hodder Education, an Hachette UK Company,
338 Euston Road, London NW1 3BH

http://www.hoddereducation.com

British Library Cataloguing in Publication Data
A catalogue record for this book is available from the British Library

Library of Congress Cataloging-in-Publication Data
A catalog record for this book is available from the Library of Congress

ISBN   978 0 340 96875 8

1 2 3 4 5 6 7 8 9 10

Commissioning Editor: Joanna Koster
Project Editor: Francesca Naish
Production Controller: Karen Tate
Cover Designer: Amina Dudhia
Indexer: Laurence Errington

Typeset in 10/12 Optima by Macmillan Publishing Solutions
(www.macmillansolutions.com)
Printed & bound in India

What do you think about this book? Or any other Hodder Arnold title?
Please visit our website: www.hoddereducation.com

To Laine, Kooks and Benjo

CONTENTS

Contents

PREFACE

Paediatrics is a fascinating and multifaceted speciality. As well as dealing with the standard medical conditions that arise in children, it covers neonatology and the pre-term infant (often newcomers to a neonatal intensive care unit see it as 'another world'), genetics, ethics, child development, child protection, and child and adolescent psychiatry. During the short medical student paediatric attachments, and in the era of decreasing hours of work for junior doctors, the exposure to the diverse range of paediatric conditions is limited.

In the 100 cases that follow, we have tried to cover the majority of the key areas in paediatrics. We have tackled problems that arise in different settings, such as primary care, and emergency departments, paediatric outpatients, the paediatric ward and the maternity and neonatal intensive care units. We hope to have done so in a way that is interesting and that brings the cases alive. After reading through the case and questions, the reader should carefully consider their answer and ideally commit their thoughts to paper, prior to looking at the answers over the page. We have also tried to demonstrate how a senior paediatrician would approach and work their way through the clinical problem and to explain some underlying principles in a way that will help cement understanding and knowledge.

The book is aimed at medical students, foundation year doctors doing paediatrics and junior doctors studying for their MRCPCH. We hope that these cases will be enjoyable and that they will keep the 'grey cells' stimulated!

J E Raine
A J Cunnington
J M Walker
October 2008

ACKNOWLEDGEMENTS

The authors would like to thank Drs Ed Broadhurst and Natasha Kapur from the Whittington Hospital, Drs Rachael Harrison and Roy Sievers from Portsmouth Hospitals NHS Trust, Mr Pat Malone from Southampton University NHS Trust and Dr Joanna Danin from Imperial College Healthcare NHS Trust.

ABBREVIATIONS

ABC	airway, breathing, circulation
A and E	accident and emergency
ALSG	Advanced Life Support Group
ALT	alanine aminotransferase
ALP	alkaline phosphatase
ANA	anti-nuclear antibody
APLS	Advanced Paediatric Life Support
ASOT	anti-streptolysin O titre
AXR	abdominal X-ray
BCG	Bacillus Calmette–Guérin
BMI	body mass index
BP	blood pressure
CNS	central nervous system
CPAP	continuous positive airways pressure
CPR	cardiopulmonary resuscitation
CRP	C-reactive protein
CSF	cerebrospinal fluid
CT	computed tomography
CXR	chest X-ray
ECG	electrocardiogram
ED	emergency department
EEG	electroencephalogram
ESR	erythrocyte sedimentation rate
FBC	full blood count
FSH	follicle-stimulating hormone
fT4	free thyroxine
GCS	Glasgow Coma Score
GP	general practitioner
HCG	human chorionic gonadotrophin
HIV	human immunodeficiency virus
IO	intraosseous
LFT	liver function test
LH	luteinizing hormone
LHRH	luteinizing hormone-releasing hormone
LP	lumbar puncture
M,C+S	microscopy, culture and sensitivity
MCV	mean cell volume
MDI	metered dose inhaler
MCH	mean corpuscular haemoglobin
MRI	magnetic resonance imaging
MSU	midstream urine
NAI	non-accidental injury

NG	nasogastric
NAD	no abnormality detected
PCR	polymerase chain reaction
PEFR	peak expiratory flow rate
PICU	paediatric intensive care unit
p.r.n.	as required
RAST	radioallergosorbent test
SLE	systemic lupus erythematosus
TB	tuberculosis
TFT	thyroid function test
TSH	thyroid-stimulating hormone
U+Es	urea and electrolytes
URTI	upper respiratory tract infection
US	ultrasound
UTI	urinary tract infection
WBC	white blood cells

NORMAL VALUES

NORMAL VALUES	

Respiratory rate at rest

Age (years)	Respiratory rate (breaths/min)
<1	30–40
1–2	25–35
2–5	25–30
5–12	20–25
>12	15–20

Heart rate

Age (years)	Heart rate (beats/min)
<1	110–160
1–2	100–150
2–5	95–140
5–12	80–120
>12	60–100

Systolic blood pressure

Age (years)	Systolic blood pressure (mmHg)
<1	70–90
1–2	80–95
2–5	80–100
5–12	90–110
>12	100–120

(Reproduced with kind permission of the Advanced Life Support Group from *Advanced Paediatric Life Support*, Blackwell Publishing, 2005.)

RESPIRATORY

CASE 1: AN INFANT WITH NOISY BREATHING

History

Mohammed is a 3-month-old boy, brought to a paediatric rapid referral clinic because of persistent noisy breathing. He was born in the UK at term after an uneventful pregnancy and is the fifth child of non-consanguineous Somalian parents. His birth weight was 3.7 kg (75th centile). Since he was a few weeks old, he has had noisy breathing, which hasn't affected his feeding, and his parents were repeatedly reassured that it would get better. He has continued to have intermittent noisy breathing, especially when agitated, and sometimes during sleep. Over the last few days, his breathing has been noisier than usual. Otherwise he has been well without any fevers. All of his siblings have recently had coughs and colds.

Examination

He is active and smiles responsively. Oxygen saturations are 95 per cent in air and his temperature is 36.9°C. He is coryzal and has intermittent stridor. There is a small 'strawberry' haemangioma on his forehead. Respiratory rate is 45/min, there is subcostal recession and mild tracheal tug. Air entry is symmetrical in the chest, with no crackles or wheeze. Cardiovascular examination is unremarkable. His weight is 6.7 kg (75th centile).

Questions
- What is the most likely cause of his stridor?
- What other important diagnoses need to be considered?
- How can the diagnosis be confirmed?

ANSWER 1

Stridor is an inspiratory sound due to narrowing of the upper airway. Mohammed is most likely to have stridor due to laryngomalacia. This means that the laryngeal cartilage is soft and floppy, with an abnormal epiglottis and/or arytenoid cartilages. The larynx collapses and narrows during inspiration (when there is a negative intrathoracic pressure), resulting in inspiratory stridor. It is usually a benign condition with noisy breathing but no major problems with feeding or significant respiratory distress. Most cases resolve spontaneously within a year as the larynx grows and the cartilaginous rings stiffen. The reason Mohammed now has respiratory distress is that he has an intercurrent viral upper respiratory tract infection.

A very important diagnosis to consider in this boy is a haemangioma in the upper airway. The majority of haemangiomas are single cutaneous lesions, but they can also occur at other sites and the upper airway is one position where they can enlarge with potentially life-threatening consequences. The presence of one haemangioma increases the likelihood of a second one. This boy should be referred for assessment by an ENT surgeon.

There are many other possible congenital causes of stridor which affect the structure or function of the upper airway. Infectious causes of stridor, such as croup and epiglottitis, are very rare in this age group.

Differential diagnosis of stridor in an infant
- Laryngomalacia
- Laryngeal cyst, haemangioma or web
- Laryngeal stenosis
- Vocal cord paralysis
- Vascular ring
- Gastro-oesophageal reflux
- Hypocalcaemia (laryngeal tetany)
- Respiratory papillomatosis
- Subglottic stenosis

The diagnosis of laryngomalacia can be confirmed by visualization of the larynx using flexible laryngoscopy. This can be done by an ENT surgeon as an outpatient procedure. This demonstrates prolapse over the airway of an omega-shaped epiglottis or arytenoid cartilages. Congenital structural abnormalities may also be seen. Lesions below the vocal cords may require bronchoscopy, CT or an MRI scan for diagnosis.

 KEY POINTS

- The commonest cause of congenital stridor is laryngomalacia.
- Laryngomalacia can be exacerbated by intercurrent respiratory infections.

CASE 2: A CHILD WITH NOISY BREATHING

History
Ewa is a 4-year-old child who presents to the ED with a sudden onset of noisy breathing. She has had a runny nose for 2 days, a cough for 1 day and developed noisy breathing 3 hours earlier. Her mother feels that she is getting progressively more breathless. Her father had a cold the previous week. She is otherwise well but has troublesome eczema which is treated with emulsifiers and steroid creams. Her mother states that she is allergic to peanuts, as they lead to a deterioration of the eczema within 1–2 hours. She avoids peanuts and all types of nuts. She is fully immunized. Her 8-year-old sister has asthma.

Examination
Oxygen saturation is 89 per cent in air. Her temperature is 38.0°C. There is loud noisy breathing, mainly on inspiration. Her respiratory rate is 52/min with supracostal and intercostal recession. On auscultation, there are no crackles or wheezes. There are no other signs.

Questions
- What is the most likely diagnosis?
- What is the differential diagnosis?
- What is the treatment?

ANSWER 2

The most likely diagnosis is laryngotracheobronchitis (croup). This child has stridor, which is an inspiratory sound secondary to narrowing of the upper airway. In contrast, wheeze is an expiratory sound caused by narrowing of the lower airways. The effort required to shift air through the narrowed airway has resulted in tachypnoea and recession.

The upper airway of a child with stridor should not be examined and the child should not be upset by performing painful procedures such as blood tests. This is because there is a small risk that this may lead to a deterioration, causing partial obstruction to progress to complete obstruction and a respiratory arrest.

! **Differential diagnosis of acute stridor**

- Laryngotracheobronchitis
- Inhaled foreign body
- Anaphylaxis
- Epiglottitis
- Rare causes include:
  - Bacterial tracheitis
  - Severe tonsillitis with very large tonsils
  - Inhalation of hot gases (e.g. house fire)
  - Retropharyngeal abscess

Croup typically occurs in children aged 6 months to 5 years. It is characterized by an upper respiratory tract infection that is followed by a barking-type cough, a hoarse voice, stridor and a low-grade fever. Croup is most commonly caused by the parainfluenza virus.

When a foreign body is inhaled, there is usually a history of sudden coughing and/or choking in a child that was previously well. There may be accompanying cyanosis. The foreign body is usually a food (e.g. peanut) but may be a small toy. On examination there may be a unilateral wheeze with decreased air entry on one side.

This case is not typical of anaphylaxis, in that there is no history of the child having had peanuts. Nor are there features that often accompany anaphylaxis, such as an itchy urticarial rash, facial swelling, vomiting, wheeze or hypotension.

Epiglottitis would be very unlikely in a fully immunized child who would have received the *Haemophilus influenzae* vaccine.

Initial management deals with the ABC. As the oxygen saturation is low, high-flow 100 per cent oxygen will be needed to elevate the saturation to ≥95 per cent.

The first step in the treatment of croup is oral dexamethasone. A less frequently used alternative is nebulized budesonide. If 2–3 hours later the child has improved and the oxygen saturation is ≥95 per cent in air, the child can be discharged. In some cases a further dose of steroids can be administered 12–24 hours later. If the child deteriorates then nebulized adrenaline can be administered. If adrenaline is required then senior help and an anaesthetist should be summoned urgently. If the child deteriorates further (increasing tachypnoea, recession and exhaustion) then intubation and ventilation are required to secure the airway and to prevent hypoxia and its sequelae. If intubation is unsuccessful, an ENT surgeon will be required to perform an emergency tracheostomy.

KEY POINTS

- Stridor is due to upper airway obstruction.
- The upper airway of a child with stridor should not be examined as this may precipitate total obstruction.
- Laryngotracheobronchitis is the commonest cause of acute stridor.

CASE 3: A CHESTY INFANT

History
Max is a 3-month-old boy seen in the community by his GP. He developed a runny nose and bit of a cough 2 days ago but has become progressively more chesty and has now gone off his feeds and is having far fewer wet nappies. He has two older siblings who also have colds. He was born at 34 weeks' gestation but had no significant neonatal problems and went home at 2 weeks of age. Both parents smoke but not in the house. His mother had asthma as a child.

Examination
Max is miserable but alert. His airway is clear. He is febrile (37.8°C) and has copious clear nasal secretions and a dry wheezy cough. His respiratory rate is 56 breaths/min with tracheal tug and intercostal and subcostal recession. On auscultation, there are widespread fine crackles and expiratory wheeze. The remainder of the examination is unremarkable.

Questions
- What is the most likely diagnosis?
- What is the commonest causative organism?
- What are the indications for referral to hospital?
- What is the management in hospital?

ANSWER 3

This baby has the characteristic clinical features of acute bronchiolitis – a seasonal viral illness occurring from early autumn to spring, principally affecting infants.

The commonest causative organism is respiratory syncytial virus (RSV), which is responsible for about 80 per cent of infections. In hospital, a nasopharyngeal aspirate (NPA) may be sent for viral immunofluorescence, polymerase chain reaction (PCR) or culture. This is largely for infection control and epidemiology and does not affect acute management.

Around 2–3 per cent of all infants are admitted each year with RSV-positive bronchiolitis but many more are managed at home. Prevention is possible with monoclonal RSV immuno-globulin (Palivizumab) but this is reserved for high-risk infants, e.g. oxygen-dependent survivors of prematurity, as it is extremely expensive. There is no immunization.

! **Indications for hospital referral**

- Apnoeic episodes (commonest in babies <2 months and may be the presenting feature)
- Intake <50 per cent of normal in preceding 24 hours
- Cyanosis
- Severe respiratory distress – grunting, nasal flaring, severe recession, respiratory rate >70/min
- Congenital heart disease, pre-existing lung disease or immunodeficiency
- Significant hypotonia, e.g. trisomy 21 – less likely to cope with respiratory compromise
- Survivor of extreme prematurity
- Social factors

Babies usually deteriorate over the first 48–72 hours. Hence there is a low threshold for admitting any baby <2 months of age on day 1–2 of their illness as they may deteriorate and become exhausted and apnoeic.

Management is supportive. Investigations are rarely indicated apart from an NPA. A chest X-ray is only needed if the clinical course is unusual and often leads to unnecessary antibiotic prescriptions. Blood tests are only required if there is diagnostic uncertainty, e.g. if the infant has a temperature ≥39°C and a superadded bacterial respiratory infection is suspected. Oxygen saturations should be kept at ≥92 per cent and the infant should be nasogastrically fed if they cannot maintain >50 per cent of normal intake. Intravenous fluids are used in severe cases. All fluids are restricted to two-thirds of maintenance. Nasal and oral suction is helpful. There is no evidence that broncho-dilators, oral or inhaled steroids modify the clinical course or any important outcomes such as the need for ventilation or the length of stay. A capillary blood gas should be checked if the infant is deteriorating. Every season a small proportion of infants need high-dependency or intensive care – most respond well to continuous positive airways pressure (CPAP), avoiding the need for intubation.

Babies are discharged when they are well enough to continue recovering at home but many continue to cough and wheeze for weeks and get similar symptoms with subsequent upper respiratory tract infections. Response to conventional asthma treatment is variable. Leukotriene antagonists may have a role. Exposure to tobacco smoke must be avoided.

 KEY POINTS

- Bronchiolitis is a clinical diagnosis.
- Numerous well-conducted studies have shown no benefit from any drug intervention in the acute phase or in the prevention of long-term sequelae.
- Monoclonal RSV immunoglobulin (Palivizumab) may be given for prevention to high-risk infants, but the costs of widespread use outweigh the benefits.

CASE 4: A CHRONIC COUGH

History

Donna is a 12-year-old girl seen in the GP surgery with her mother. This is her fourth visit in 3 months. Her initial presentation was with a headache, fever, malaise, a sore throat and a symmetrical non-pruritic rash on her arms and hands. The lesions varied in size and character, some being simple red macules and others being up to 2 cm in diameter with a central, slightly dusky centre and a surrounding 'halo' of varying erythema. A diagnosis of a viral infection was made. However, these symptoms progressed to include a cough productive of white sputum. The computer records show that the emergency GP they consulted at the time heard some crackles throughout the chest and prescribed a course of clarithromycin. All of her symptoms have resolved, except for her cough. This is mostly during the day and is not waking her or her family. However, it is disrupting her life because she is being sent home from school and her parents have excluded her from sport. It is a spasmodic unproductive cough that comes in bouts, which are occasionally severe enough to cause vomiting. Another GP gave her a trial of inhaled salbutamol but with no apparent improvement. She has never had any obvious nasal symptoms. Donna is otherwise well and recently started her periods. She is fully immunized. Her father has a history of asthma. Her mother smokes but 'not around the children'. There is no history of recent foreign travel and no family history or contact with tuberculosis.

Examination

Donna looks well. Her height is on the 91st centile and her weight is on the 75th centile. There has been appropriate weight gain since her illness began. She is not clubbed or anaemic. She is afebrile. There is no significant lymphadenopathy. Examination of the ears, nose and throat is normal. Her pulse is 72 beats/min, her heart sounds are normal and there are no murmurs. Inspection of the chest is normal and her respiratory rate is 18 breaths/min. Expansion, percussion and auscultation are normal. Examination of the abdomen is unremarkable.

🔍 INVESTIGATIONS	
Full blood count	Normal
C-reactive protein	Normal
Erythrocyte sedimentation rate	Normal
Chest X-ray 6 weeks previously	Normal

Questions
- What is the differential diagnosis?
- What is the most likely diagnosis?
- What was the rash?
- What is the management?

ANSWER 4

Cough is one of the commonest symptoms in childhood and indicates irritation of nerve receptors within the airway.

! **Differential diagnosis of a recurrent or persistent cough in childhood**

- Recurrent viral URTIs – very common in all age groups but more so in infants and toddlers
- Asthma – unlikely without wheeze or dyspnoea
- Allergic rhinitis – often nocturnal due to 'post-nasal drip'
- Chronic non-specific cough – probably post-viral with increased cough receptor sensitivity
- Post-infectious – a 'pertussis (whooping cough)-like' illness can continue for months following pertussis, adenovirus, mycoplasma and chlamydia
- Recurrent aspiration – gastro-oesophageal reflux
- Environmental – especially smoking, active or passive
- Suppurative lung disease – cystic fibrosis or primary ciliary dyskinesia
- Tuberculosis
- Habit

Donna is otherwise healthy with no evidence of any chronic disease and she has a normal chest X-ray. Although her father has asthma, she has no convincing features of atopy and she did not respond to inhaled salbutamol. The history is not that of recurrent aspiration. The abrupt onset of symptoms with systemic features suggests infection, and the description of her cough as spasmodic bouts with occasional vomiting is that of a 'pertussis-like' illness. This can continue for months following an infection, as can a chronic, non-specific cough following a viral infection.

The acute history is very typical, although not specific, for *Mycoplasma pneumoniae* infection. This aetiology is supported by the rash, which has the characteristic clinical features of erythema multiforme (EM). As expected from the name, EM has numerous morphological features but the diagnosis is made on finding the classic target-like papules with an erythematous outer border, an inner pale ring and a dusky purple to necrotic centre. It is occasionally mistaken for urticaria, but EM is largely asymptomatic and the lesions do not fade within 24 hours. Infection, frequently mycoplasma, is one of numerous causes. No treatment is indicated.

These symptoms cause understandable distress and anxiety and a belief that there must be something wrong and that treatment is necessary. As in this case, children must have a thorough clinical evaluation to exclude serious and treatable pathology. This, plus an explanation that they can expect the cough to take months to resolve, is usually adequate to reassure families. Explore the reasons behind their anxiety and encourage a return to normality knowing that no harm is being done. A watch-and-wait policy is best, resisting any pressure to investigate further or to try other treatments such as inhaled steroids. The one thing the family can do is to ban smoking in the house and this could be the spur for her mother to give up altogether.

KEY POINTS

- Cough is one of the commonest symptoms in childhood and is usually due to viral respiratory tract infections.
- A chronic cough may indicate a serious disorder and all such children should have a thorough clinical review to exclude significant pathology.

CASE 5: RECURRENT CHEST INFECTIONS

History

Conor is a 4-year-old boy who is admitted to the paediatric ward from the A&E department with pneumonia. This is his fourth hospital admission. In the first year of life, he was admitted twice with bronchiolitis, requiring several days on oxygen, and about 6 months ago he was admitted with pneumonia, again requiring oxygen and intravenous antibiotics. He has had many courses of oral antibiotics over the last few years from his GP for chest infections. He also has recurrent abdominal pain and his parents report large offensive stools. His parents both smoke 20–30 cigarettes/day. He is unimmunized as his parents are worried about potential side-effects.

Examination

He is small (height ninth centile, weight second centile), pale-looking, miserable and very clingy to his mother. He has finger clubbing. His temperature is 38.7°C, respiratory rate 40 breaths/min, heart rate 140 beats/min and oxygen saturation 89 per cent in air (95 per cent in facemask oxygen). There is reduced air entry at the left base with bronchial breath sounds in the left midzone, and coarse crackles are heard on both sides of the chest. Cardiovascular examination is unremarkable. His abdomen is mildly distended but non-tender.

INVESTIGATIONS		
		Normal
Haemoglobin	10.1 g/dL	11.0–13.8 g/dL
White cell count	19.7×10^9/L	6–17×10^9/L
Platelets	401×10^9/L	210–490×10^9/L
Immunoglobulin G	10.2 g/L	5.0–15.0 g/L
Immunoglobulin A	2.5 g/L	0.3–3.0 g/L
Immunoglobulin M	1.8 g/L	0.4–2.0 g/L
Chest radiograph – see Figure 5.1		

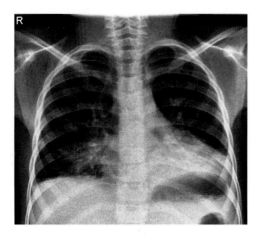

Figure 5.1 Conor's chest radiograph.

Questions
- What does the chest radiograph show?
- What is the likely underlying diagnosis?
- What investigation would you do to confirm the diagnosis?
- What are the other manifestations of this disease?

ANSWER 5

The chest radiograph shows consolidation with some collapse of the left lower lobe and further consolidation in the right middle lobe. There are small bilateral pleural effusions. These features are consistent with the clinical diagnosis of pneumonia.

The combination of clubbing and recurrent chest infections is strongly suggestive of cystic fibrosis (CF). This is the commonest cause of clubbing in children in the UK. Normal immunoglobulins exclude antibody deficiencies such as X-linked hypogammaglobulinaemia. Malabsorption (with bulky, offensive stools) is another common feature of CF.

Cystic fibrosis is an autosomal recessive condition affecting 1 in 2500 children born in the UK. It is the commonest autosomal recessive disorder in the Caucasian population. Cystic fibrosis is caused by defects in the gene for the CF transmembrane conductance regulator (CFTR). This gene encodes for a protein that functions as a chloride channel and is regulated by cyclic AMP. Cystic fibrosis causes dysfunction of multiple organs – most prominently lung, intestine, pancreas and liver. Clinical phenotypes of CF can be very variable, affecting the age at presentation, symptoms and the severity of different organ involvement. Thus CF should be considered in any of the situations listed below.

! Presentations of cystic fibrosis

Neonatal
- Meconium ileus
- Intestinal atresia
- Hepatitis/prolonged jaundice

Infant
- Rectal prolapse (may be recurrent)
- Failure to thrive
- Malabsorption and vitamin deficiency (A, D, E, K)

Older children
- Recurrent chest infections
- 'Difficult' asthma
- Haemoptysis
- Nasal polyps
- Distal intestinal obstruction syndrome
- Liver disease
- Diabetes mellitus

Diagnosis can be made by the sweat test, which will demonstrate elevated sweat sodium and chloride concentrations, and by genetic testing. National newborn screening using blood spots collected on day 5 of life are now tested for immunoreactive trypsinogen (at the same time as testing for phenylketonuria, congenital hypothyroidism and sickle cell disease). This is now leading to the identification of cases before the onset of clinical disease.

Once a child is diagnosed with CF, he or she will need multidisciplinary team management under the supervision of a paediatric respiratory consultant. Optimal care will aim to maintain lung function by treating respiratory infections and removing mucus from the airways with physiotherapy, and to maintain adequate growth and nutrition with pancreatic enzyme and nutritional supplements.

KEY POINTS

- Cystic fibrosis should be considered in children with recurrent chest infections or malabsorption.
- Cystic fibrosis is the commonest cause of finger clubbing in children.

CASE 6: A WHEEZY TEENAGER

History

Bradley is a 13-year-old boy who is seen in the A&E department at the request of the GP out-of-hours service. He is a known asthmatic and this is his third attendance with an acute wheeze in 3 months. His mother reports that last time he was nearly transferred to the paediatric intensive care unit (PICU). He has developed a cold and become acutely breathless and is using his salbutamol inhaler hourly without much relief. The accompanying letter says that he is prescribed a beclometasone metered dose inhaler (MDI) 100 μg/metered inhalation 2 puffs b.d., salmeterol MDI 50 μg/metered inhalation 1 puff b.d. and salbutamol MDI 100 μg/metered inhalation p.r.n.

Examination

Bradley is sitting up in bed with a nebulizer in progress containing 5 mg salbutamol. His oxygen saturation on 15 L of oxygen on arrival is documented as 89 per cent. He is quiet but able to answer questions with short sentences. His chest is hyperinflated (increased anteroposterior diameter) and he is using his accessory muscles of respiration. His respiratory rate is 60 breaths/min and he has marked tracheal tug with intercostal and subcostal recession. On auscultation there is equal but poor air entry with widespread expiratory wheeze. His temperature is 37.6°C. His pulse is 180 beats/min with good perfusion.

Questions

- What is the most likely underlying cause for this acute episode?
- What signs would you look for of impending respiratory failure?
- Outline your management plan for this acute episode
- What should happen before he is discharged?

ANSWER 6

This boy has another acute exacerbation of asthma. Much the most likely underlying cause is poor adherence to home treatment. This is common in all age groups but particularly in teenagers with their growing independence and risk-taking behaviour.

! Signs of impending respiratory failure

- Exhaustion (this is a clinical impression)
- Unable to speak or complete sentences
- Colour – cyanosis ± pallor
- Hypoxia despite high-flow humidified oxygen
- Restlessness and agitation are signs of hypoxia, especially in small children
- Silent chest – so little air entry that no wheeze is audible
- Tachycardia
- Drowsiness
- Peak expiratory flow rate (PEFR) persistently <30 per cent of predicted for height (tables are available) or personal best. Children <7 years cannot perform PEFR reliably and technique in sick children is often poor

---

Acute management goals are to correct hypoxia, reverse airway obstruction and prevent progression. Reassurance and calm are crucial because he will be frightened. Give high-flow oxygen via mask and monitor saturations. Start a regular inhaled β-agonist (e.g. salbutamol) via a nebulizer. Beta-agonists can be given continuously. If so, cardiac monitoring is needed as side-effects include irritability, tremor, tachycardia and hypokalaemia. Inhaled ipratropium bromide can be added. Give oral prednisolone or intravenous (IV) hydrocortisone. Frequent clinical review is paramount. Blood gases (capillary or venous) and a chest X-ray may be required. If there is no improvement or the child deteriorates, additional treatment is needed. These include IV salbutamol, IV magnesium sulphate (a smooth muscle relaxant) and IV aminophylline, although the effectiveness of the latter two is still controversial. His precipitating 'cold' is almost certainly viral and antibiotics are unlikely to be beneficial.

Before discharge a thorough review of his asthma is needed:

- How often does he miss his regular drugs?
- Is there parental supervision?
- What device does he use? Children rarely use MDIs effectively and need a spacer. However, he is unlikely to use one because they are cumbersome and not 'cool'. Agree an alternative 'breath-activated' device with the proviso that, if acutely wheezy, he must use a spacer.
- Consider changing to a combined steroid/long-acting β-agonist inhaler. This should improve adherence.
- Ask about smoking – him and his family. Adults should be encouraged to stop smoking or to smoke outside.
- Educate about allergen avoidance, e.g. daily vacuuming to reduce house dust mites. Consider measuring total IgE and specific allergen IgE (RAST) if the history suggests allergies.
- All asthmatics should have a written home management plan.

- Provide an asthma symptom diary and arrange hospital follow-up until control improves. Most children can and should be managed in primary care. Primary care and hospital-based asthma specialist nurses are very helpful.

KEY POINTS

- The commonest cause of an acute deterioration in chronic asthma is poor adherence to treatment.
- Home management should be reviewed during any acute admission.

CASE 7: FEVER AND BREATHLESSNESS

History
Niall is a 3-year-old boy from a travelling family referred to the paediatric day unit by the out-of-hours GP service. He was seen 4 days ago with a cough and fever and diagnosed with a viral upper respiratory tract infection (URTI). The following day he returned and was commenced on oral antibiotics. He is now complaining of tummy ache and has vomited once. The GP is worried that he is becoming dehydrated and may have a urinary tract infection or intra-abdominal pathology. He has not been immunized but there is no other medical history of note.

Examination
Niall is miserable, flushed, toxic and febrile (38.8°C) with a capillary refill time of 2 s. His pulse is 140 beats/min, his oxygen saturation is 91 per cent in air and his blood pressure is 85/60 mmHg. He seems to be in pain, especially when he coughs, and his respiratory rate is 48 breaths/min with nasal flaring. There is dullness to percussion in the right lower zone posteriorly with decreased breath sounds and bronchial breathing. He seems reluctant to have his abdomen examined but bowel sounds are normal.

INVESTIGATIONS		
		Normal
Haemoglobin	11.8 g/dL	11.5–15.5 g/dL
White cell count	25.4×10^9/L	$6–17.5 \times 10^9$/L
Neutrophils	20.8×10^9/L	$3–5.8 \times 10^9$/L
Platelets	467×10^9/L	$150–400 \times 10^9$/L
Sodium	126 mmol/L	138–146 mmol/L
Potassium	3.5 mmol/L	3.5–5.0 mmol/L
Urea	2.5 mmol/L	1.8–6.4 mmol/L
Creatinine	48 µmol/L	27–62 µmol/L
Glucose	4.5 mmol/L	3.3–5.5 mmol/L
C-reactive protein	387 mg/L	<6 mg/L
Chest X-ray – see Figure 7.1		

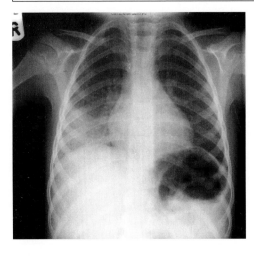

Figure 7.1 Niall's chest X-ray.

Questions

- What are the chest X-ray findings?
- What is the most likely causative organism?
- What complication may have arisen and how would you confirm it?
- List the steps in management.

ANSWER 7

The chest X-ray shows loss of the right hemidiaphragm, right lower zone consolidation and a normal right heart border – the characteristic features of right lower lobe pneumonia. Lower lobe pneumonia should always be on the list of differential diagnoses for abdominal pain in children. Young children rarely localize pain but observation should establish whether they have pleuritic pain – they may have shallow breathing or may simply sit very still, hardly moving the affected side.

The most likely causative organism is *Streptococcus pneumoniae*. However, a diagnosis is rarely made from sputum analysis because children tend to swallow their sputum. Blood cultures may be positive. Children in the UK are immunized against *Streptococcus pneumoniae* but not all strains are covered, there is emerging antibiotic resistance and also 'failed' immunizations. Any immunized child with positive cultures should be investigated for an underlying immune problem, including an absent spleen.

Niall has hyponatraemia. There are no pointers to excess sodium loss (e.g. diarrhoea or significant vomiting) and hence the most likely cause is the syndrome of inappropriate antidiuretic hormone secretion (SIADH), a known association with pneumonia. The hyponatraemia is dilutional. First, the result should be confirmed – taking blood from children can be difficult and unexpected results should be repeated. At the same time, urine should be sent for osmolality and sodium. His serum osmolality is calculated as follows:

$$2 \times ([Na] + [K]) + [urea] + [glucose] = 266\,mosmol/kg\ (normal\ 278-305)$$

Normally a fall in serum osmolality would suppress antidiuretic hormone secretion to allow excretion of excess water as dilute urine. In SIADH, urine osmolality is inappropriately high (>320 mosmol/kg) and urine sodium is usually >40 mmol/L (unlike hypovolaemic states where it is <20 mmol/L).

! Steps in management

- Oxygen to maintain saturation at >92 per cent
- Adequate pain relief for pleuritic pain
- Intravenous antibiotics according to local guidelines, e.g. co-amoxiclav
- Initial fluid restriction to two-thirds maintenance to help correct the hyponatraemia. Fluid restrict even if no hyponatraemia, as SIADH may still develop
- Fluid balance, regular urea and electrolytes – adjust fluids accordingly. Weigh twice daily
- Physiotherapy, e.g. bubble blowing. Encourage mobility
- Monitor for development of a pleural effusion. If the chest X-ray is suspicious, an ultrasound will be diagnostic. If present, a longer course of antibiotics is recommended to prevent empyema (a purulent pleural effusion). A chest drain may be necessary if there is worsening respiratory distress, mediastinal shift on the chest X-ray, a large effusion or failure to respond to adequate antibiotics
- Ensure adequate nutrition – children have often been anorectic for several days. Low threshold for supplementary feeds probably via nasogastric tube
- Organise immunization programme before discharge
- Arrange a follow-up chest X-ray in 6–8 weeks for those with lobar collapse and/ or an effusion. If still abnormal, consider an inhaled foreign body

KEY POINTS

- A lower lobe pneumonia should always be considered in the differential diagnosis of an acute abdomen in children.
- 'Vaccine failures' should be investigated for an underlying immune problem.

CASE 8: A TEENAGER WITH CHEST PAIN

History

Fabio is a 13-year-old boy who presents to outpatients with a 6-month history of chest pain. The pain can occur at rest or on exercise and is central with no radiation. It lasts for up to an hour. He occasionally gets palpitations after exercise, which he describes as regular. The pain is not accompanied by light-headedness and he has never fainted. He has no respiratory or gastrointestinal symptoms. He had asthma as a child and has a salbutamol inhaler at home but has had no symptoms in the past few years. There is a family history of hypertension and his grandfather died of a myocardial infarction a year ago.

Examination

His pulse is 86/min, regular, his blood pressure is 124/82 mmHg and his heart sounds are normal. There is no hepatomegaly. Femoral pulses are palpable and his chest is clear. His peak expiratory flow rate (PEFR) is 460 L/min (child's height 1.62 m, PEFR range 320–570 L/min). On palpation there is no chest tenderness.

INVESTIGATIONS
His ECG and chest X-ray are both normal.

Questions
- What is the most likely diagnosis and the differential diagnosis?
- What treatment would you suggest?

ANSWER 8

The most likely diagnosis in this case is idiopathic chest pain. This is one of the commonest causes of chest pain in children. Psychological chest pain, which may be a replication of the pain his grandfather used to have, and may be secondary to various stresses such as bullying, is a further possibility. Costochondritis is due to inflammation of the cartilage that connects the inner end of each rib with the sternum. There may be tenderness on palpation of the cartilage in the anterior chest wall and the pain may be worse on movement or coughing. The cause is unknown and the condition is self-limiting.

The lack of respiratory symptoms and signs with the normal PEFR would go against a respiratory cause. PEFR is related to height, and charts with normal values exist. Children have to be 5 or more years of age in order to perform this test in an effective and consistent manner, and normally the best reading out of three is obtained. Pneumonia with pleurisy is a common cause of chest pain that is typically worse on inspiration. In the case of a pneumothorax, the pain is sudden and associated with shortness of breath. A severe cough from whatever cause can lead to musculoskeletal chest pain.

The lack of gastrointestinal symptoms such as vomiting would go against gastro-oesophageal reflux. Cardiac disease is a rare cause of chest pain in children. The palpitations described are probably secondary to tachycardia during exercise.

!	**Differential diagnosis of chest pain**

- Trauma, e.g. fractured rib
- Exercise, e.g. overuse injury
- Idiopathic
- Psychological, e.g. anxiety
- Costochondritis
- Pneumonia with pleural involvement
- Asthma
- Severe cough
- Pneumothorax
- Reflux oesophagitis
- Sickle cell disease with chest crisis and/or pneumonia
- *Rare*: pericarditis, angina, e.g. from severe aortic stenosis, osteomyelitis, tumour

The patient and his family should be reassured. Ibuprofen could be used on an as necessary basis for its analgesic and anti-inflammatory properties for the more prolonged bouts of pain. The child should be reviewed in about 2 months to monitor progress.

KEY POINTS

- Chest pain in children is often idiopathic, psychological or musculoskeletal in origin.
- Pulmonary causes are a further common cause of chest pain.
- Cardiac disease is a rare cause of chest pain in children.
- A chest X-ray and ECG should be done to rule out significant pathology.

CARDIOLOGY

CASE 9: A CYANOSED NEWBORN

A 5-hour-old male newborn on the postnatal ward is noticed by the midwife because he looks blue around the lips and tongue. He is the first child of a 27-year-old mother with asthma who was taking inhaled steroids throughout pregnancy. Antenatal scans were unremarkable. She went into spontaneous labour at 41 weeks and there was thin meconium staining of the liquor when the membranes ruptured 1 hour before delivery. Cardiotocograph monitoring during labour revealed normal variability of fetal heart rate. The baby was born by normal vaginal delivery and weighed 3.3 kg. The Apgar scores were 7 at 1 min and 8 at 5 min.

Examination

The baby is not dysmorphic. His temperature is 36.6°C and his central capillary refill time is 2 s. His lips, tongue and extremities are cyanosed. He is crying normally and has no signs of increased respiratory effort. Heart rate is 160 beats/min, femoral pulses are palpable, heart sounds are normal and no murmur is audible. Oxygen saturation is 70 per cent in air and does not rise with facial oxygen, which has been administered by the midwife. There is no hepatosplenomegaly.

INVESTIGATIONS		
Arterial blood gas	*Normal*	
In air		
pH	7.25	7.35–7.42
Pa_{O_2}	4.7 kPa	9.3–13.3 kPa
Pa_{CO_2}	5.0 kPa	4.7–6.0 kPa
After 10 min in high-flow facemask oxygen		
pH	7.23	7.35–7.42
Pa_{O_2}	5.3 kPa	9.3–13.3 kPa
Pa_{CO_2}	5.2 kPa	4.7–6.0 kPa

Questions
- What is the likely diagnosis and differential diagnosis?
- How do you interpret the blood gas results?
- What is the emergency management?

ANSWER 9

This baby is most likely to have transposition of the great arteries. There are few congenital cyanotic heart conditions that present on the first day of life, because in most cases the ductus arteriosus remains open at this stage, maintaining pulmonary blood flow in conditions such as pulmonary and tricuspid atresia where pulmonary blood flow would be severely restricted or absent. Severe Ebstein's anomaly and obstructed total anomalous pulmonary venous drainage can produce early cyanosis, but these conditions are associated with significant respiratory distress. Persistent fetal circulation also results in cyanosis, usually with respiratory distress in the context of a newborn who has suffered a significant hypoxic, hypothermic or hypoglycaemic insult, who has pulmonary hypoplasia or sepsis, or sometimes for unknown reasons.

Transposition of the great arteries accounts for up to 5 per cent of congenital heart disease and is the commonest cardiological cause of cyanosis in the newborn. The aorta and pulmonary arteries are transposed such that the right ventricle delivers deoxygenated blood, returning from the systemic circulation, into the aorta and back to the systemic circulation. The left ventricle delivers oxygenated blood, arriving from the lungs, into the pulmonary arteries and back to the lungs. These two parallel circulations would result in the vital organs never receiving oxygenated blood, and hence rapid death, if it was not for mixing in the atria via the foramen ovale and between the aorta and pulmonary arteries via the ductus arteriosus. Chest X-ray may show a narrowed upper mediastinum due to the abnormal position of the aorta and pulmonary arteries. Echocardiography by an experienced operator is necessary to confirm the diagnosis.

The hyperoxia test provides a means of diagnosing whether cyanosis is due to cardiac or respiratory disease. Normally arterial $P_a O_2$ is greater than 9 kPa and rises to more than 20 kPa after exposure to 90–100 per cent oxygen. If the $P_a O_2$ fails to rise, this is strongly suggestive of cyanotic heart disease. Persistent fetal circulation can also result in a lack of response. There is already evidence of tissue hypoxia in this case, as there is a metabolic acidosis.

Emergency management involves commencing a prostaglandin infusion to maintain patency of the ductus arteriosus, and to correct the metabolic acidosis. An emergency balloon atrial septostomy will probably be needed to improve mixing of oxygenated and deoxygenated blood at the atrial level. Ultimately, an arterial switch operation will need to be performed to provide an anatomical correction.

 KEY POINTS

- Measure oxygen saturations if you have any suspicion that a baby may be cyanosed.
- The absence of a murmur does not exclude congenital heart disease.

CASE 10: A SHOCKED NEONATE

History

Freddie is 3 days old. He is brought by ambulance to the resuscitation room in A&E. He was found in his cot this morning looking mottled and breathing very fast. He had been well until yesterday when he did not feed as well as usual. He was born at 39 weeks' gestation by normal vaginal delivery in a midwife-led birthing unit and was discharged home the same day. There was no prolonged rupture of membranes and he did not require any resuscitation at birth. He has been exclusively breast-fed. He did not receive vitamin K due to parental objection.

Examination

Freddie is grunting and has a respiratory rate of 70/min with subcostal, intercostal and sternal recession. His lung fields sound clear. Oxygen saturation monitoring does not pick up a trace. He looks mottled, cyanosed peripherally and his limbs feel cold. Capillary refill time is 5s, heart rate is 180/min, blood pressure is unrecordable, and the femoral pulses cannot be felt. The heart sounds are unremarkable. The liver edge is palpable 3 cm below the costal margin and his temperature is 35.0°C.

INVESTIGATIONS		
		Normal
Arterial blood gas		
pH	7.01	7.35–7.42
$Paco_2$	5.3. kPa	4.7–6.0 kPa
Pao_2	8.1 kPa	9.3–13.3 kPa
HCO_3	10 mmol/L	18–20 mmol/L
Base excess	−18	+2.5 to −2.5 mmol/L
Glucose	3.8 mmol/L	3.3–5.5 mmol/L

Questions
- What is the interpretation of the blood gas result?
- What is the most likely diagnosis and what is the differential?
- What is the initial management of a collapsed neonate?

ANSWER 10

The pH is 7.01, which is a severe acidosis. The $Paco_2$ is normal, so the acidosis is not respiratory in origin. The low bicarbonate and large negative base excess indicate that this is a metabolic acidosis. There is also a degree of hypoxaemia. The baby's circulation is so poor that pulses are not palpable, the saturation meter cannot pick up a pulse trace and a severe metabolic acidosis has developed due to hypoperfusion.

This is most likely to be a case of cardiogenic shock due to a congenital left heart obstructive lesion. The clues are in the age of the baby and the absence of the femoral pulses. Left-sided obstructive cardiac lesions rely on the ductus arteriosus to perfuse the systemic circulation by passage of blood from the pulmonary arteries into the distal end of the aortic arch. As the ductus arteriosus closes, the systemic perfusion becomes dramatically reduced, resulting in collapse and shock. Freddie actually had hypoplastic left heart syndrome (HLHS). The absence of a murmur does not rule out a cardiac cause, and murmurs are not always present in HLHS.

! **Congenital cardiac lesions presenting with neonatal collapse**

- Severe aortic coarctation
- Aortic arch interruption
- Hypoplastic left heart syndrome
- Critical aortic stenosis

! **Differential diagnosis of a collapsed neonate**

- Infection – e.g. group B *Streptococcus*, herpes simplex
- Cardiogenic – e.g. hypoplastic left heart syndrome, supraventricular tachycardia
- Hypovolaemic – e.g. dehydration, bleeding
- Neurogenic – e.g. meningitis, subdural haematoma ('shaken baby')
- Lung disorder – e.g. congenital diaphragmatic hernia (late presentation)
- Metabolic – e.g. propionic acidaemia, methylmalonic acidaemia
- Endocrine – e.g. panhypopituitarism

In any collapsed neonate, it is essential to adopt a standard approach to resuscitation. The airway should be maintained, high-flow oxygen administered, intravenous access obtained and fluid resuscitation should be given for the shock. Blood glucose measurement must be checked early and corrected if low. A blood gas sample should be analysed. Intravenous antibiotics should be given promptly as sepsis is a possible treatable cause. If there is any suspicion of a duct-dependent cardiac lesion, a prostaglandin infusion should be commenced, as this is life-saving. Early involvement of senior paediatricians, an anaesthetic team and paediatric intensive care services will help appropriate management.

 KEY POINTS

- Congenital cardiac disease can present as shock in a neonate after several days.
- The absence of a murmur does not rule out congenital heart disease.
- A prostaglandin infusion can maintain patency of the ductus arteriosus and can be life-saving.

CASE 11: A PALE, BREATHLESS BABY

History

Alfie is a 7-month-old baby who is seen in the A&E department with a day's history of pallor. Over the past few hours, he has also become restless and breathless. He is feeding poorly. He has no cough or wheeze. There is no past medical history of note and he is on no medication. His 3-year-old sister has a cold but a 5-year-old brother and the rest of the family are well.

Examination

He is apyrexial, pale and his oxygen saturation is 91 per cent in air. The heart rate is 270 beats/min, blood pressure is 84/44 mmHg, heart sounds are normal and femoral pulses are palpable. The peripheral capillary refill is 4 s. Respiratory rate is 62 breaths/min and the chest is clear. The liver is palpable 4 cm below costal margin. There are no other signs.

INVESTIGATIONS		
		Normal
Haemoglobin	12.8 g/dL	10.5–13.5 g/dL
White cell count	7.0×10^9/L	$4.0–11.0 \times 10^9$/L
Platelets	323×10^9/L	$150–400 \times 10^9$/L
Sodium	138 mmol/L	135–145 mmol/L
Potassium	3.9 mmol/L	3.5–5.0 mmol/L
Urea	6.4 mmol/L	1.8–6.4 mmol/L
Creatinine	60 μmol/L	20–80 μmol/L
C-reactive protein	5 mg/L	<6 mg/L
ECG – see Figure 11.1		

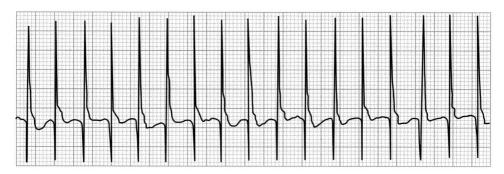

Figure 11.1 Alfie's electrocardiogram (lead 2).

Questions

- What does the ECG show and what is the diagnosis?
- What treatments can be used to manage this condition?

ANSWER 11

The ECG shows a narrow QRS complex tachycardia with a rate of approximately 220 beats/min. There are no P waves.

The diagnosis is supraventricular tachycardia (SVT). This is the commonest pathological arrhythmia in childhood (sinus arrhythmia is a normal variant). Diagnosis is based on the presence of a narrow QRS complex tachycardia. P waves are only visible in about half of cases. It is usually secondary to a re-entrant tachycardia using an accessory pathway. It is also associated with the Wolff–Parkinson–White syndrome (see Fig. 11.2). This condition can be diagnosed by a short PR interval and a slow upstroke of the QRS (delta wave). These are normally only seen when the patient does not have a tachycardia.

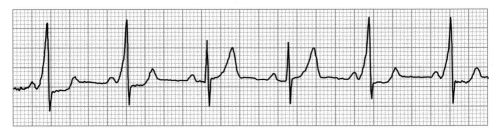

Figure 11.2 Intermittent pre-excitation in Wolff–Parkinson–White syndrome. The first two beats show the short PR interval and delta wave. The middle two beats are normal and the abnormality returns in the final two beats. (Reproduced with permission from Worrell DA, ed, *Oxford Textbook of Medicine*, 2003, Oxford University Press.)

The heart rate in SVT is typically 200–300 beats/min. Arrhythmias can last from a few seconds to days. In older children, they can be associated with palpitations, light-headedness and chest discomfort. However, in young infants, the inability to report symptoms may lead to presentation with heart failure and shock, as in this case. In a third of cases there is associated congenital heart disease so an echocardiogram should be performed. Supraventricular tachycardia needs to be differentiated from sinus tachycardia. In the latter, the heart rate is usually <220 beats/min, there is greater variability in the heart rate and there is often a history consistent with shock.

!	**Features of heart failure**
	• Tachycardia
	• Tachypnoea
	• Hepatomegaly
	• Poor feeding
	• Sweating
	• Excessive weight gain (acutely)
	• Poor weight gain (chronically)
	• Gallop rhythm
	• Cyanosis
	• Heart murmur

Initial treatment in this emergency follows the standard resuscitation guidelines and the baby should be administered oxygen. Capillary refill is slightly prolonged but should improve swiftly following the correction of the tachycardia.

Specific treatment comprises vagal stimulation, for instance by eliciting the 'diving reflex' which will increase vagal tone, slow atrioventricular conduction and abort the tachycardia. This can be done by placing a rubber glove filled with iced water over the baby's face. If this fails, the baby's face can be immersed in iced water for 5 s. Second-line treatment comprises intravenous adenosine that can be administered in escalating doses. If this fails, synchronized DC cardioversion will almost always stop the tachycardia. Once sinus rhythm is achieved, maintenance treatment using drugs such as amiodarone should be started following consultation with a cardiologist. Infants (<1 year old) with SVT are less likely to relapse than older children. They are often treated for 1 year, following which the medication is slowly tapered. In the majority of cases, the SVT does not recur. Definitive treatment comprises catheterization with radiofrequency ablation.

 KEY POINTS

- SVT is the commonest pathological arrhythmia in childhood.
- It can lead to heart failure and shock.
- Treatments comprise vagal manoeuvres, adenosine and DC cardioversion.

CASE 12: AN INCIDENTAL MURMUR

History

Lola is a 3-year-old girl referred to outpatients by her GP, who heard a murmur when she presented to him with a fever and a cough. Looking through her notes, the murmur was not heard at her 6-week check and she has only been seen twice since, with minor infections. He brought her back a week later to listen again, the murmur was still present and he has referred her on. She is otherwise entirely healthy with no significant past medical or family history.

Examination

Lola looks generally healthy and her height and weight are on the 75th centiles. She is not clinically anaemic, jaundiced or cyanosed. Her pulse is 88/min and her blood pressure 90/50 mmHg. She has normal femoral pulses. Examination of the praecordium shows no thrills but there is a heave at the lower left sternal border. The apex beat is in the fifth inter-costal space in the mid-clavicular line. Both heart sounds are present but the pulmonary component of the second sound is quiet. There is a click immediately after the first heart sound and an ejection systolic murmur which is heard loudest in the pulmonary area. This radiates into both lung fields and is heard in the back between the scapulae. Examination of the respiratory and abdominal systems is normal with no hepatomegaly.

🔍	INVESTIGATIONS
	Lola's electrocardiogram is shown in Figure 12.1.

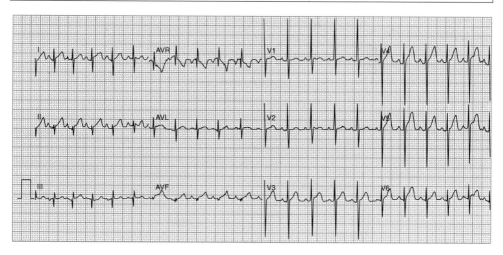

Figure 12.1 Lola's electrocardiogram.

Questions

- Why did the GP bring her back to listen again?
- What features suggest that a murmur is innocent?
- What is the most likely diagnosis?
- What does the ECG show?
- What should happen next?

ANSWER 12

Up to 40 per cent of children will have a murmur heard at some time during childhood, particularly if examined at a time of high cardiac output – e.g. fever, anaemia or anxiety. These 'innocent' murmurs have certain reassuring features and the heart is structurally normal. It is good practice to re-examine asymptomatic healthy children 1–2 weeks later when they are well. If the murmur persists, they should be referred. That it was not heard at the 6-week check is irrelevant – murmurs in children are often difficult to hear. A murmur can be diagnosed as innocent on the basis of the certain clinical findings (see box).

! **Clinical findings in innocent murmurs**

- Asymptomatic
- No thrills or heaves
- Normal heart sounds, normally split with no added clicks
- Quiet and soft
- Systolic (isolated diastolic murmurs are never innocent)
- Short, ejection (pansystolic murmurs are pathological)
- Single site with no radiation to neck, lung fields or back
- Varies with posture (decreases or disappears when patient sits up, loudest when they're lying)

Further investigations are rarely indicated. Nevertheless parents are understandably anxious and must be reassured that an innocent murmur is simply a 'noise'. It may never disappear but this does not matter because the heart is normal. All other murmurs should be investigated. However, a normal ECG and chest X-ray do not exclude pathology. An echocardiogram is the definitive test.

The findings are characteristic of moderate pulmonary valve stenosis (PS). This is common, accounting for 7–10 per cent of all congenital heart defects. Unless the stenosis is severe, children are otherwise healthy and asymptomatic. An 'opening' click may be heard at the beginning of systole. With increasing severity, the clinical features change to reflect the progressive narrowing and the resulting right ventricular hypertrophy (RVH). The pulmonary component of the second heart sound diminishes and a lower left sternal heave develops. In severe PS there may be evidence of right-sided heart failure with hepatomegaly.

The ECG will show the same progression. This child's ECG shows right axis deviation and evidence of RVH (an 'R' in V1 > 20 millimetres, an 'S' in V6 > 5 millimetres and upright T waves across all the right precordial leads).

She needs an echocardiogram to:

- confirm the clinical diagnosis
- assess severity to guide further investigation and treatment
- exclude any associated cardiac lesions, e.g. ventricular septal defect.

Doppler echocardiography measures velocity across the valve – the higher this is, the greater the need for intervention. Catheter balloon valvuloplasty is the treatment of choice in the majority and the outcomes are good. Milder degrees of PS need regular re-evaluation to monitor any progression. Antibiotic prophylaxis to prevent infective endocarditis is no longer recommended in this condition.

 KEY POINTS

- Cardiac murmurs are heard at some time in up to 40 per cent of children.
- The majority of murmurs in children are innocent.
- A normal ECG and chest X-ray do not exclude a pathological murmur.
- An echocardiogram is the definitive investigation.

CASE 13: A FUNNY TURN

Sian is a 15-year-old girl, referred to paediatric outpatients by her GP. The letter says, 'Thank you for seeing this girl who has had her first fit.' Three weeks ago she was at school when the fire alarm went off unexpectedly. She felt faint and clammy. Friends tried to help her to walk out of the classroom, but after about a minute she collapsed to the floor and had a brief episode of jerking movements affecting all four limbs. There was no incontinence or tongue biting. She regained consciousness within a minute but continued to feel weak for a few hours afterwards.

Sian had a febrile convulsion at 18 months of age and she has fainted on about five occasions, mostly in emotional situations or when it has been hot. She describes herself as an anxious girl, and has a sensation of her heart racing every few weeks. She has never been in hospital, but has seen her GP for heavy periods. There is no family history of epilepsy, but her aunt collapsed and died at the age of 28 in Canada. She is top of her year at school and hopes to be a doctor or lawyer.

Examination

Her height is 170 cm (91st centile) and her weight is 53kg (50th). Cardiovascular, respiratory, abdominal and neurological examinations are normal.

Questions
- What are the possible causes of her collapse?
- What is the most important investigation to perform at this stage?

ANSWER 13

> **!** **Causes of a funny turn**
>
> | | Distinguishing features in the history |
> |---|---|
> | Epileptic seizure | Aura, incontinence, tongue biting, family history |
> | Cardiac arrhythmia | Palpitations, sudden collapse, exercise-related |
> | Neurally mediated syncope | Preceding stimulus, dizziness, nausea |
> | Panic attack | Hyperventilation, paraesthesia, carpopedal spasm |
> | Breath-holding attack | Usually a toddler, upset/crying |
> | Reflex anoxic seizure | Usually infant/toddler, painful stimulus |
> | Pseudoseizures | Psychological problems |
>
> *Other causes*
> Hypoglycaemia
> Other metabolic derangements
> Drugs, alcohol

In this case, the history is most suggestive of a neurally mediated (vasovagal) syncope, a cardiac arrhythmia or perhaps a panic attack. The history is less typical of an epileptic seizure, and the most likely reason for the brief convulsion is hypoperfusion of the brain due to low blood pressure while her friends held her upright – an anoxic seizure. This terminated quickly when she was supine after collapsing.

The single most important investigation is an ECG, as this may show a potentially life-threatening cardiac cause. An EEG is generally not performed after a first seizure because it may be normal in those who go on to have epilepsy and abnormal in those who never have another seizure, with the EEG adding little to prognosis at this stage. Blood tests are often performed for glucose, electrolytes, calcium and magnesium, but are frequently unhelpful. Sian's ECG is shown in Figure 13.1.

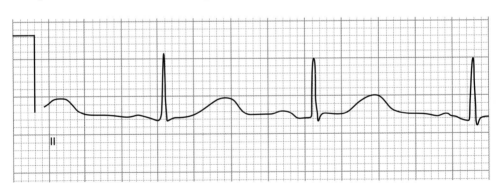

Figure 13.1 Sian's electrocardiogram.

Her ECG shows a prolonged corrected QT interval, making the diagnosis of a long QT syndrome. This disorder has a number of genetic causes, and in some cases an arrhythmia can be precipitated by a sudden loud noise. This girl went on to require anti-arrhythmic drug treatment and an implantable cardiodefibrillator.

The QT interval is measured from the start of the QRS complex to the end of the T-wave; the QT interval is corrected (QTc) for heart rate by: QTc = QT/($\sqrt{R - R}$ interval). QTc is normally around 0.41 s and should be less than 0.45 s. In this case it is 0.52 s.

KEY POINTS

- The commonest cause of fainting in a teenager is neurally mediated (vasovagal) syncope.
- Cardiac causes should always be considered in the differential of epilepsy and funny turns.
- An ECG is almost always indicated.

ENDOCRINOLOGY AND DIABETES

CASE 14: A THIRSTY BOY

History

Steven is a 4-year-old boy seen in the paediatric day unit with a 2-week history of polydipsia and polyuria. Having been dry at night for some time, he has also started wetting the bed. His mother thinks that he has lost some weight. He has been less cheerful than usual and hasn't wanted to go to school – his mother has put this down to tiredness at the end of his first term. She and her mother have hypothyroidism. There is no significant past medical history and he is fully immunized. He has a 2-year-old brother who is well.

Examination

Steven is playing happily in the playroom. His weight is on the 9th centile and his height is on the 50th centile. His trousers are a bit loose round his waist. He is afebrile. He is not dehydrated. His pulse is 84 beats/min and his capillary refill time is <2s. Examination of the respiratory and abdominal systems is normal.

INVESTIGATIONS		
		Normal
Haemoglobin	12.3 g/dL	11.5–15.5 g/dL
White cell count	8.4×10^9/L	$6–17.5 \times 10^9$/L
Platelets	365×10^9/L	$150–400 \times 10^9$/L
Sodium	138 mmol/L	138–146 mmol/L
Potassium	4.5 mmol/L	3.5–5.0 mmol/L
Urea	4.2 mmol/L	1.8–6.4 mmol/L
Creatinine	46 µmol/L	27–62 µmol/L
Glucose	22.4 mmol/L	3.3–5.5 mmol/L
Venous blood gas		
pH	7.35	7.35–7.45
P_{CO_2}	4.3 kPa	4.7–6.4 kPa
Bicarbonate	19 mmol/L	22–29 mmol/L
Urinalysis	Glucose +++, ketones +++	

Questions

- What is the diagnosis?
- What should happen next?
- List the topics that need to be discussed with his family?

ANSWER 14

The diagnosis is type 1 diabetes mellitus (T1DM), by far the commonest form of diabetes in childhood characterized by pancreatic β-cell dysfunction with insulin deficiency. The precise mechanism is not understood, but environmental factors probably 'trigger' a T-cell-mediated autoimmune process in those genetically susceptible (although only about 10 per cent have a family history at presentation). There may be a history of other autoimmune diseases. The incidence is rising. The incidence of type 2 is also rising alongside obesity.

Although this boy has ketonuria, he is not acidotic and does not have diabetic ketoacidosis (DKA) – a widely accepted biochemical definition being a pH <7.30 and/or a bicarbonate <15 mmol/L. Nor is he vomiting or showing signs of sepsis. Therefore he does not need intravenous fluids or intravenous insulin. Only about 10–20 per cent of children present with DKA, usually pre-school children in whom the diagnosis has not been considered. Childhood DKA has a mortality rate of approximately 0.2 per cent, usually from cerebral oedema due to the use of excessive fluids and/or rapid changes in blood glucose.

He now needs to start regular subcutaneous insulin. Current best practice suggests that insulin is best delivered by a 'basal bolus' regime – background 'basal' insulin given once daily with rapid-acting 'bolus' insulin at mealtimes. Alternatives are twice-daily injections of pre-mixed long and rapidly acting insulins or insulin via a pump.

The impact of the diagnosis of T1DM should never be underestimated (see Case 87, p. 255 in relation to the breaking of bad news to families). At diagnosis, he and his family will start a detailed education programme. Education is provided by a multidisciplinary team, including specialist nurses and dieticians. The aspects of management that need to be discussed include:

- how to give insulin – to a probably reluctant 4-year-old
- regular finger-prick blood testing – up to four times daily
- interpreting blood glucose results and altering insulin
- recognition and treatment of hypoglycaemia – 'hypos' really worry parents and older patients, especially at night
- management during intercurrent illness, e.g. flu
- blood or urine ketone estimations
- who to contact in an emergency
- diet – matching insulin to carbohydrate in a 'basal-bolus' regime
- school – trusting staff in everyday care
- peer group relationships – diabetes risks making children feel 'different'
- exercise
- the 'honeymoon' period
- long-term complications – discuss even at outset because many families know about and fear complications and need objective information
- using glycosylated haemoglobin (HBA1c) to measure overall control
- membership of local and/or national support groups.

KEY POINTS

- The cardinal features of type 1 diabetes are polydypsia and polyuria.
- Most patients do not present in DKA.
- Patients with DKA are acidotic (pH < 7.30) as well as having ketonuria.
- Education and support from a multidisciplinary specialist team are crucial.

CASE 15: A TALL BOY

History

Zak is a 10-year-old boy referred to outpatients by his GP with tall stature. He is seen with his 28-year-old mother who is not particularly concerned because his 29-year-old father is 1.93 m, although he does not come from a tall family himself. However, friends and family have begun to comment and the parents are seeking reassurance. When asked, the boy admits that he is self-conscious about his stature and is fed up with being treated as older than his true age. At school, everyone expects him to take more responsibility than he thinks is fair. He is otherwise healthy although he was seen in infancy with a cardiac murmur that was thought to be innocent. He did not have an echocardiogram. He is doing well academically at school. His 7-year-old sister is apparently on the 75th percentile for height. His mother is measured in clinic and is 1.66 m tall. This puts her between the 50th and 75th centiles for a female.

Examination

Zak is tall and slender. His height is 1.58 m (>99.6th centile) and weight 35 kg (75th centile). His arm span is 168 cm. He has long, tapering fingers and his thumb, when completely opposed within the clenched hand, projects beyond the ulnar border. He has pectus excavatum (funnel chest) but an otherwise normal respiratory examination. He has a midsystolic click with a late systolic murmur heard at the apex. Examination of the abdomen is normal and he is prepubertal.

Questions

- What is the most likely diagnosis?
- What further investigations does he need?
- Who else should be examined and by whom?

ANSWER 15

The most likely diagnosis is the connective tissue disease Marfan syndrome. This is an inherited synthetic disorder of fibrillin-1, a glycoprotein constituent of the microfibrils of elastic fibres that anchor non-elastic tissue such as the aortic adventitia and the suspensory ligament of the eye.

By definition, tall stature includes all children with a length or height above the 98th centile. However, uncovering pathology in such children is rare and the vast majority have simple familial tall stature. This is characterized by a normal physical examination and serial height measurements that show no growth acceleration. Skeletal age (assessed by a bone age X-ray of the wrist) is usually slightly advanced in relation to chronological age, the child enters puberty relatively (not abnormally) early and completes their growth phase relatively early, with a final height within the expected range for their family. The differential diagnosis of familial tall stature is a syndrome associated with tall stature, such as Marfan or Klinefelter (47, XXY) syndrome, or a child with growth acceleration for which an endocrine cause is likely, e.g. sexual precocity, thyrotoxicosis or growth hormone excess. Children with familial tall stature rarely benefit from further investigations or monitoring.

The diagnosis of Marfan syndrome is made on accepted clinical criteria – only about 60–70 per cent of patients who fulfil these have an identifiable mutation in the fibrillin gene. This boy displays many of the musculoskeletal features – arm span to height ratio >1.05, arachnodactyly with a positive thumb sign and pectus excavatum – but many other systems may be involved. Most important are the eyes and heart. Lens dislocation is one of the major criteria for diagnosis and he needs a slit-lamp examination. His murmur is typical of mitral valve prolapse (MVP) and echocardiography is essential for diagnosis and to monitor the high risk of progressive aortic root dilatation.

Marfan syndrome is an autosomal dominant disorder, although about 30 per cent arise sporadically. There is the distinct possibility that this boy has inherited it from his father, who is unusually tall for his family and should be investigated. There is significant morbidity and reduced longevity, mainly from the cardiovascular complications, but young adults like him may still be asymptomatic. However, making such a diagnosis will have far-reaching social, financial and psychological consequences for an individual and their family. Referral to the genetics team is mandatory: first, to obtain informed consent for investigations; second, to confirm the diagnosis; and third, to counsel about recurrence and inheritance risk – in Marfan this is 50 per cent. Refuting a diagnosis is obviously just as important in uncertain cases and the geneticists are best placed to do so.

KEY POINTS

- Pathological causes of tall stature are rare.
- Families who may have serious inheritable disorders must be referred to genetics teams for diagnosis and counselling.

CASE 16: A SHORT GIRL

History

Tanya is a 4-year-old girl brought to the GP by her mother, who is worried about her daughter's growth. She has noticed that her shoe size has not changed for almost 12 months and she is still in clothes for a 2- to 3-year-old. She was born at 38 weeks by normal delivery and weighed 2.1 kg (<9th centile). Her mother tried breast-feeding but she was never easy to feed, even with a bottle. She is generally healthy, apart from recurrent ear infections that have needed grommet insertion. She wears glasses for long-sightedness. Her development is normal, although nursery staff have reported that she seems to have poor concentration.

Examination

She is generally healthy and certainly well nourished. The GP notices wide-spaced nipples and a low hairline but can find no other obvious abnormalities. She creates a growth chart from her own and the mother's records (Fig. 16.1).

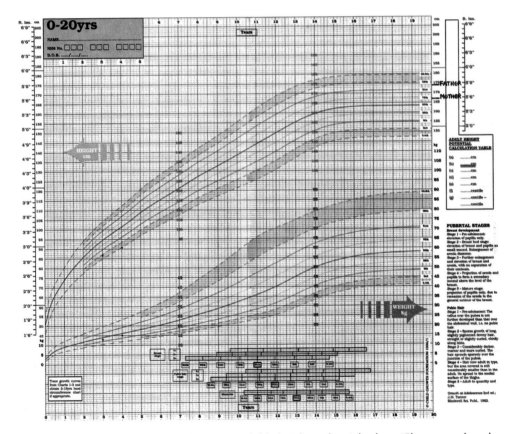

Figure 16.1 Tanya's growth chart showing available height and weight data. (Chart reproduced with kind permission of the Child Growth Foundation.)

Questions

- How did the GP plot the parents' heights?
- What are the clinical signs that suggest a pathological cause for short stature?
- What is the most likely diagnosis?

ANSWER 16

Plotting the parents' centiles establishes whether a child falls into the expected height range for their family. Both parents should be measured, but realistically this is often difficult. To plot the father's centile on a girls' chart, 14 cm is subtracted from his height, and on a boys' chart the same measurement is added to the mother's height. Alternatively, their centile is taken from the relevant chart. The 'target centile range' can also be calculated. This is the midpoint of the two plotted parental centiles ±8.5 cm for a girl and ±10 cm for a boy. With normal parents and healthy children, final heights will be normally distributed within these 95 per cent confidence limits.

Growth is unique to childhood and an excellent tool for confirming health as well as spotting disease. Children who are healthy grow and gain weight normally and follow centiles. The challenge in assessing a short child is to pick out those with a pathological cause from the majority without. Usually there is no one defining feature and pieces of the clinical jigsaw are put together from the history, examination, growth pattern and any investigations. A short child following the 0.4th to 2nd centiles from a short family is less worrying than one who is crossing the centiles downwards due to abnormally slow growth. The causes are numerous – chronic disease (coeliac disease, uncontrolled asthma), drug effects (steroids), endocrine disorders (hypothyroidism, growth hormone deficiency) and emotional abuse. Thorough clinical assessment is crucial.

! **Clinical signs suggesting a pathological cause for short stature**

- Extreme short stature – on or below 0.4th centile.
- Short for family size – outside target range for parents
- Short and relatively overweight – suggests an endocrinopathy
- Short and very underweight – suggests poor nutrition ± malabsorption
- Growth failure – crossing the centiles downwards
- Dysmorphic features
- Skeletal disproportion – charts available for ratio between sitting height and leg length. Significant disproportion suggests a skeletal dysplasia, e.g. achondroplasia
- Signs of systemic disease, e.g. clubbing

This girl is extremely short, crossing the centiles, short for family and has some subtle dysmorphic features. Pathology is probable. She is also relatively overweight for height, suggesting an endocrinopathy. The GP should refer her to a growth clinic.

The most likely diagnosis is Turner syndrome (TS) caused by the complete or partial absence of one of the X chromosomes. The incidence is 1 in 3000 live female births. Short stature is universal and there are specific Turner growth charts. The dysmorphic features vary in frequency (e.g. only 50 per cent have neck webbing) and are often subtle. This girl has wide-spaced nipples and a low hairline. She also has some of the other associations – low birth weight, difficult to feed in infancy, middle ear disease, visual problems and poor concentration. None of these are specific, but put together they make TS likely. Investigations must include chromosome analysis.

  KEY POINTS

- Most children seen with short stature do not have a pathological cause.
- Dysmorphic features in Turner syndrome may be subtle and there should be a low threshold for chromosome analysis in all short girls.

CASE 17: AN OVERWEIGHT BOY

History

Marlon is a 7-year-old boy who presents to paediatric outpatients because he's overweight. His father became concerned 1 year ago. His mother is overweight, hypertensive and has type 2 diabetes, but his father's weight is average. His father says the boy's diet is generally good but that his grandmother spoils him. He does sports twice a week at school. He is bullied at school about his weight. His birth weight was 3.8 kg and there were no problems in the neonatal period. He snores every night but his parents have not noticed any sleep apnoea. His development is normal. He is on no medication. No other diseases run in the family.

Examination

There are no dysmorphic features. There are some pink abdominal stretch marks. There is no acanthosis nigricans and no goitre. His blood pressure is 116/75 mmHg. His tonsils are large but with a good gap between them. There are no other signs. His height is 125 cm (75th centile) and his weight is 38.7 kg (>99.6th centile).

INVESTIGATIONS
Full blood count, urea and electrolytes, liver and thyroid function tests are normal. His fasting glucose, insulin, cholesterol and triglycerides are normal.

Questions

- What is this child's body mass index (BMI)?
- What is the most likely cause of this child's obesity?
- How should this child be treated?

ANSWER 17

Marlon's BMI = weight (kg)/height $(m)^2$ = $38.7/(1.25)^2$ = $24.8\,kg/m^2$. There are stand-ard BMI charts for males and females from 0 to 20 years. BMI varies according to age. Children with a BMI above the 91st centile are overweight and those with a BMI above the 98th centile are obese.

The most likely cause of this child's obesity is simple obesity – obesity due to caloric intake exceeding energy expenditure. It is the commonest cause of obesity and is not due to any underlying pathology. Children with simple obesity tend to be tall and over-weight. Those who are short and overweight are more likely to have underlying path-ology, such as an endocrine disorder.

Stretch marks are secondary to the obesity and are usually pink. Violaceous stretch marks are associated with Cushing's syndrome. Large tonsils and obstructive sleep apnoea are associated with obesity. The child does not have acanthosis nigricans, which is a thickening and darkening of the skin in the axilla, neck or groin. It is usually a sign of insulin resistance. Children with obesity should be assessed for co-morbidities such as hypertension, breathlessness on exertion, obstructive sleep apnoea, hyperinsulinaemia and type 2 diabetes (in children ⩾10 years), dyslipidaemia, knock-knees or bow legs, polycystic ovary syndrome and psychosocial dysfunction.

! Causes of obesity

- Simple obesity
- Genetic, i.e. one or both parents is obese
- Endocrine disease, e.g. hypothyroidism, Cushing's syndrome, growth hormone deficiency, pseudohypoparathyroidism
- Drugs, e.g. steroids, sodium valproate
- Syndromes, e.g. Down's, Präder–Willi and Laurence–Moon–Biedl
- Disorders associated with immobility, e.g. cerebral palsy
- Hypothalamic damage, e.g. secondary to trauma or brain tumours
- Rarely, single gene mutations, such as those of the melanocortin-4 receptor and leptin

---

Treatment should be multidisciplinary. Dietetic input is very important. Children should be encouraged to exercise for 60 min/day. Sedentary activities such as playing com-puter games should be discouraged. Obesity can lead to low self-esteem and, in our case, Marlon is being bullied. He would therefore benefit from seeing a psychologist, who could also initiate behavioural therapies to help treat the obesity.

As the enlarged tonsils are not leading to sleep apnoea, tonsillectomy is not currently indicated. The systolic blood pressure is below the 95th centile for a 7-year-old male with a height on the 75th centile and therefore does not need treatment.

Drug treatment with drugs such as Orlistat or sibutramine is reserved for children ⩾12 years of age and is only recommended in the presence of severe physical or psychological co-morbidities. Post-puberty, bariatric surgery, such as gastric stapling, can be considered in severe cases.

KEY POINTS

- Body mass index is calculated by weight (kg)/height $(m)^2$.
- A child with a BMI above the 91st centile is overweight and one with a BMI above the 98th centile is obese.
- The commonest cause of obesity is simple obesity.

History

Tracey is a 6.5-year-old Afro-Caribbean girl who presents to the paediatric clinic with a 1-year history of breast development and a 9-month history of pubic and axillary hair. She sweats more than previously and has body odour. She has no acne. Her periods have not started. Her mother feels that she has been growing taller at a faster rate in the past year. She has headaches but these occur less than once a month and are not severe. She has no visual problems. Her mother had her menarche at the age of 13 years. There is no past medical history of note.

Examination

Her breasts are Tanner stage 3, and her pubic hair Tanner stage 2 (see p. 60). There is sparse axillary hair. There are no neurological signs and no abdominal masses or organomegaly. Her height, at 133 cm, is just over the 99.6th centile and her weight, at 27 kg, is on the 91st centile (mid-parental height between 50th and 75th centile).

INVESTIGATIONS

Oestradiol – 172 pmol/L (prepubertal value <50)

Luteinizing hormone-releasing hormone (LHRH) test

Time (min)	Luteinizing hormone (LH, units/L)	Follicle-stimulating hormone (FSH, units/L)
0	3.8	3.0
30	14.2	7.3
60	36.4	12.6

Pelvic ultrasound – bilaterally enlarged ovaries with multiple small follicular cysts, the largest being 7 mm in diameter.
The uterus is enlarged for age. There is no endometrial stripe
Bone age – 9.5 years
Cranial MRI – see Figure 18.1

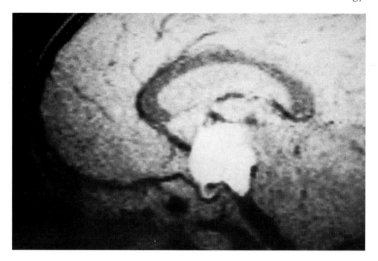

Figure 18.1 Cranial MRI. (Reproduced with permission from Raine JE, Donaldson MDC, Gregory JW *et al.*, *Practical Endocrinology and Diabetes in Children*, Blackwell Science, 2006.)

Questions

- What is the precise diagnosis?
- What is the treatment?

ANSWER 18

Tracey has gonadotrophin-dependent precocious puberty secondary to a hypothalamic hamartoma. This condition differs from gonadotrophin-independent precocious puberty, which is caused by the abnormal secretion of sex steroids independent of the hypothalamo-pituitary axis. Precocious puberty is defined in the UK as puberty commencing before the age of 8 years in females and 9 years in males. In the United States these criteria have been recently revised to below 7 years in a Caucasian girl and below 6 years in an Afro-Caribbean girl. There may be a family history.

The first sign of puberty in girls is breast development, and in boys is testicular enlargement with a testicular volume of ≥4 mL denoting the start of puberty.

Tracey's puberty started at 5 years and 6 months. Sweating, body odour, acne and a height spurt (height velocity increases from 5 cm/year prepubertally to as much as 12 cm/year) are all part of puberty. The high height centile relative to the mid-parental centile and the advanced bone age all support early puberty. The LHRH test can help diagnose gonadotrophin-dependent precocious puberty. An LH value ≥8 units/L with a predominant LH response is diagnostic. The ultrasound is also in keeping with puberty. In the majority of girls (>90 per cent) the cause is idiopathic. The earlier the onset of puberty, the greater the likelihood of there being a cause. Investigation should be considered in all girls below 8 years of age. The presence of neurological features should also prompt investigations, including a cranial MRI. In a minority of girls, a hypothalamic hamartoma can lead to early puberty. Rarely, malignant brain tumours can cause precocious puberty. Acquired neurological injuries, such as encephalitis, hydrocephalus and radiation, can also lead to early puberty.

In contrast, in boys early puberty is usually secondary to a cranial lesion and MRI scanning is mandatory.

Treatment is with monthly injections of an LHRH analogue. This should halt puberty and may lead to some regression. Although currently tall, this girl is at risk of premature fusion of her epiphysis with a short adult height. Psychosocial considerations are also an important indication for treatment. Coping with the emotional changes of puberty and possible early menarche is difficult in young girls. In girls with mild, slowly progressive early puberty, no treatment may be necessary. In boys, treatment is also with an LHRH analogue. Any underlying lesion should be treated. Treatment is often continued until 11 years of age.

Hypothalamic hamartomas are benign and often remain static in size or grow slowly, producing no other signs. Neurosurgical intervention is not indicated except in rare patients with intractable seizures.

KEY POINTS

- Precocious puberty is defined as puberty starting below the age of 8 years in girls and 9 years in boys.
- In females it is usually idiopathic, but in males it is usually secondary to a cranial lesion.
- Treatment is with LHRH analogues (any underlying lesion may also need treatment).

CASE 19: A BOY WITH DELAYED PUBERTY

History

Paul, who is 14 years and 6 months old, comes to see his GP for the first time in years. He is worried about his short stature and lack of pubertal development. He feels he is losing out in team sports and wants to become a physical education teacher. The GP records show that his father is on the 9th centile and his mother is between the 9th and 25th centiles. There are no other symptoms or past history of note.

Examination

Paul is a fit, healthy, slim boy. General and systems examination are normal. His penis is about 5 cm long and the skin of the scrotum is lax and slightly pigmented. Both testes are descended but are quite small. There is no pubic or axillary hair. Both height and weight are on the 2nd centile. The GP puts together a growth chart from the available data (see Fig. 19.1).

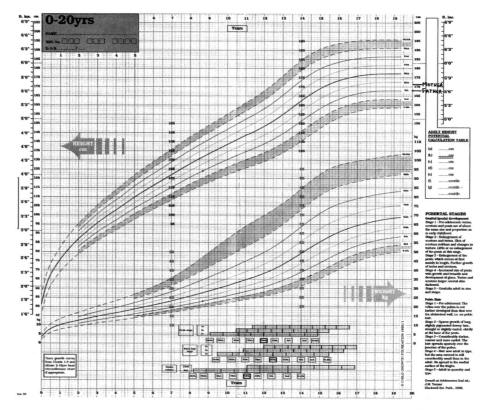

Figure 19.1 Paul's growth chart. (Chart reproduced with kind permission of the Child Growth Foundation.)

Questions

- What is the most likely diagnosis?
- What should the GP do next?
- Is there any treatment available?

ANSWER 19

The most likely diagnosis is constitutional delay of growth and puberty (CDGP) in a boy from a relatively short family. Boys enter puberty any time from 9 to 14 years old and it takes 4–5 years to complete. Puberty follows a recognized pattern with initial enlargement of the testes that produce testosterone and gradual development of secondary sexual characteristics according to Tanner stages 1 (prepubertal) to 5 (adult) – a scoring system for genital and hair development. Testicular volume can be estimated using a Prader orchidometer, 4 mL defining the onset of puberty and 15–25 mL being an adult male. This boy is only at stage 2 for genital development and stage 1 for pubic hair. Testosterone is a poor growth promoter in low concentrations (unlike oestrogen in females) so the growth spurt of puberty peaks relatively late (stage 4). Girls enter puberty between 8 and 13 years of age, hit their peak height velocity at around stage 3 and stop growing sooner than boys. Hence women are shorter than men.

Constitutional delay of growth and puberty is common in boys and can be a source of misery and behaviour problems. Boys who also come from a short family may feel very different from their peer group at a time when conforming is important. This boy's growth failure is apparent due to the current cross-sectional charts falsely depicting all boys having their growth spurt simultaneously. Unlike longitudinal charts, they take no account of the age range of normal puberty. Boys with CDGP continue to grow at their prepubertal rate, crossing the centiles downwards with later acceleration and catch-up. A family history is common. CDGP is rare in girls and a pathological cause for significant pubertal delay should be sought.

The fact that the boy has summoned the courage to seek advice means he is worried. Understandably, many give an air of bravado to cover their embarrassment. Ask about bullying and teasing. Many are satisfied with reassurance that all will be well in the end, but this boy is unlikely to start his growth spurt for 12–18 months. Unless the boy is clearly reassured, the GP should refer him to the endocrine clinic.

Treatment is usually available with a short course of low-dose, 4-weekly testosterone injections to give a 'boost' to pubertal development and thereby a growth spurt. This will have no adverse effect on final height. Usually the diagnosis is clear and no investigations are necessary except for a bone age which usually shows delay. The latter is reassuring to the family in that it demonstrates that there is additional growth potential and that the child is likely to continue to grow after his peers have stopped. If there is any uncertainty about the diagnosis, the endocrine clinic will institute further investigations.

 KEY POINTS

- Conforming to their peer group is very important for adolescents.
- Constitutional delay of growth and puberty is a rarer diagnosis in girls and a pathological cause should be sought.

CASE 20: IS IT A BOY OR A GIRL?

History

A midwife calls the neonatal intensive care unit asking for an urgent review of a baby born 10 minutes ago. At delivery they thought it was a boy and said this to the parents. Now they are not so sure because although the baby appears to have a penis, there is no obvious scrotum and they cannot feel the testes. The baby seems otherwise normal and there was nothing remarkable about the pregnancy. It is the parents' first child.

Examination

There are no dysmorphic features and examination of the cardiovascular, respiratory and abdominal systems are normal. The weight is 3.1 kg. There is a 1.5 cm phallus (normal in term newborn males ⩾2.5 cm) with a single perineal opening at the base of the phallus. There is pigmentation of the labioscrotal folds, which are fused with no obvious vaginal opening. There are no palpable gonads, including in the inguinal canals. The anus is normally positioned. The baby's external genitalia can be seen in Figure 20.1.

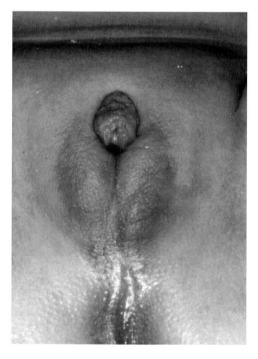

Figure 20.1 External genitalia.

Questions

- Is this a boy or a girl?
- What is the most likely diagnosis and the differential?
- What investigations are needed?

ANSWER 20

At this stage, no one can or should say whether this baby is a boy or a girl. It is impera-
tive not to guess as it could be either a virilized female (a normal girl exposed in utero
to excess androgens) or an undervirilized male. Disorders of sexual differentiation (DSD)
are a medical and social emergency and families find it exceptionally difficult not knowing the sex of their baby. Pending urgent tests they should not name the baby or register
the birth.

In the absence of palpable gonads, but with evidence of virilization with a small phallus
and pigmentation, it is most likely that this is a virilized female. Much the commonest
aetiology is congenital adrenal hyperplasia (CAH). If the baby is an undervirilized male,
there is a much larger differential, including disorders of gonadotrophin production (e.g.
Kallman syndrome), defects of testosterone synthesis and end-organ insensitivity due to
androgen receptor abnormalities. With very severe undervirilization, it is possible that
the sex of rearing should be female. Such babies need urgent referral to a specialist centre
with a team of endocrinologists, urologists, geneticists and psychologists.

Congenital adrenal hyperplasia is a group of autosomal recessive inborn errors of metabolism (IEM) (therefore commoner if parents are consanguineous), within the adrenal
steroidogenic pathways that produce mineralocorticoids (aldosterone), glucocorticoids
(cortisol) and androgens (testosterone). Ninety-five per cent of cases are due to 21-
hydroxylase deficiency (21-OHD) that catalyses late steps in the first two pathways. The
consequences are the same as for any IEM – deficiency of the end product, continued
drive through the pathway, build-up of precursors and diversion down alternative pathways. Lack of cortisol causes hypoglycaemia and a poor stress response. Elevated precursors divert to the androgen pathway and testosterone virilizes both male and female
fetuses. Most babies are also aldosterone-deficient. Those missed at birth (usually virilized boys) classically present in the second week of life with a salt-wasting (Addisonian)
crisis – vomiting and shocked with severe hyponatraemia, hyperkalaemia and acidosis.

Patients with 21-OHD need lifelong steroid replacement, initially with hydrocortisone
and fludrocortisone (a mineralocorticoid analogue), and endocrine monitoring.

The timing of any surgery to reduce clitoromegaly and create a vaginal orifice is
controversial.

Investigations in the first few days consider the differential diagnosis and monitor for
complications:

- karyotype – result in 48 hours if laboratory warned
- pelvic and abdominal ultrasound – extremely helpful and immediately available
- 17-hydroxyprogesterone – sent after 48 hours as raised in all newborns
- full male hormone profile
- urine steroid profile – confirms site of block in steroidogenic pathway
- electrolytes and glucose – from day 2; monitor bedside glucose
- plasma renin activity – best estimation of salt status.

⚷ KEY POINTS

- Never guess the sex of a newborn baby with abnormal genitalia.
- Virilization of a female infant is almost always congenital adrenal hyperplasia due to
  21-hydroxylase deficiency.

CASE 21: A BOY WITH BREASTS

History

Anthony is a 15-year-old boy who presents to an outpatient clinic with an 18-month history of gynaecomastia. There is occasional breast tenderness. There is no history of galactorrhoea. He has stopped doing sports at school as he is too embarrassed to undress in front of his classmates in the changing room. He is a little behind at school and requires extra help. His aunt has breast cancer and his grandmother died of breast cancer. He is on no medication and has no allergies.

Examination

There is moderate symmetrical gynaecomastia. Pubertal staging is as follows (see p. 60): pubic hair, Tanner stage 4; genitalia, Tanner stage 3. Testes are both 15mL in volume (using the Prader orchidometer). There are no abdominal masses and no other signs.

His weight, at 78kg, is between the 91st and 98th centiles and his height, at 169cm, is on the 50th centile.

INVESTIGATIONS		
		Normal
Follicle-stimulating hormone	2.9 units/L	1.8–10.6 units/L
Luteinizing hormone	3.3 units/L	0.4–7.0 units/L
Testosterone	9.2 nmol/L	7.6–21.5 nmol/L
Oestradiol	98 pmol/L	30–130 pmol/L

Questions

- What is the diagnosis?
- What is the treatment?

ANSWER 21

Anthony has pubertal gynaecomastia. All males have small amounts of oestrogen, just as all females have small amounts of adrenal androgens (which, in females, leads to the development of pubic and axillary hair). Gynaecomastia is common in pubertal males and is due to a decreased ratio of testosterone to oestrogen in puberty.

Klinefelter's syndrome (XXY) can be associated with gynaecomastia and learning difficulties. These patients also have small testes and this makes that diagnosis unlikely in our patient. Gynaecomastia is occasionally familial. Very rarely, oestrogen-secreting tumours can lead to gynaecomastia, e.g. a feminizing adrenal tumour or a Leydig cell tumour of the testis. The absence of abdominal signs, of a unilaterally enlarged testis and the normality of the oestradiol level make these diagnoses very unlikely. Drugs such as oestrogen and spironolactone and drugs of abuse, such as marijuana, can also cause gynaecomastia.

Prolactinomas are not usually accompanied by gynaecomastia and the absence of galactorrhoea makes this diagnosis unlikely. Breast cancer would be exceptionally rare in puberty.

Mild-to-moderate cases of pubertal gynaecomastia need no investigation. The condition is transient and usually lasts for several months to 2 years. Anthony is somewhat overweight and a proportion of the breast enlargement could be accounted for by adipose rather than breast tissue. Advice on weight loss could therefore be helpful. In mild-to-moderate cases, reassurance usually suffices. If the gynaecomastia is severe, or is leading to psychosocial problems, e.g. severe teasing, plastic surgery is indicated. Mammary reduction by either liposuction or a subareolar incision with removal of the excess tissue can be performed.

 KEY POINTS

- Gynaecomastia is common in pubertal boys.
- Reassurance usually suffices, but occasionally plastic surgery is indicated.

CASE 22: A BOY WITH BOW LEGS

History

Tariq is a 2-year-old Asian boy who presents to paediatric outpatients with bow legs and poor weight gain. He was born in Bangladesh and the family moved to the UK when he was 3 months old. He was breast-fed for the first year. His mother states that he currently has several bottles of cow's milk a day and that he has a poor appetite with a poor intake of solids. He has no gastrointestinal symptoms. His mother feels that he is not as active as other boys his age. There is no history of fractures. There is no family history of note.

Examination

His is pale, with a prominent forehead and a marked bow leg deformity. He has swollen wrists (see X-ray in Fig. 22.1) and ankles. There are no other clinical signs. His height is on the 25th centile, and his weight is on the 2nd centile.

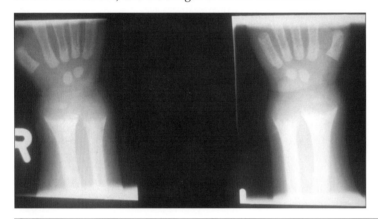

Figure 22.1 Tariq's wrist X-ray.

INVESTIGATIONS

		Normal
Haemoglobin	9.8 g/dL	11.5–15.5 g/dL
Mean cell volume	64 fL	70–86 fL
Mean corpuscular haemoglobin	22 pg	24–30 pg
White cell count	8.7×10^9/L	$4.0–11.0 \times 10^9$/L
Platelets	572×10^9/L	$150–400 \times 10^9$/L
Ferritin	4 ng/mL	15–200 ng/mL
Haemoglobinopathy screen	Normal	
Sodium	137 mmol/L	135–145 mmol/L
Potassium	4.1 mmol/L	3.5–5.0 mmol/L
Urea	4.7 mmol/L	1.8–6.4 mmol/L
Creatinine	60 μmol/L	27–62 μmol/L
Calcium	2.21 mmol/L	2.20–2.70 mmol/L
Phosphorous	1.30 mmol/L	1.25–2.10 mmol/L
Alkaline phosphatase (ALP)	1372 U/L	145–420 U/L
Bilirubin	16 μmol/L	2–26 μmol/L
Alanine aminotransferase (ALT)	32 U/L	10–40 U/L

Questions

- Name the two disorders that affect this child.
- What is the treatment?

ANSWER 22

This type of nutritional history in an Asian child, the accompanying clinical signs, the high ALP, the borderline calcium and the wrist X-ray all point to rickets. Furthermore, the poor nutritional intake, the pallor and the microcytic hypochromic anaemia are typical of iron deficiency anaemia.

Rickets is a disorder characterized by a failure in the mineralization of growing bones. The majority of cases are due to inadequate sunlight exposure coupled with nutritional deficiency. The condition is more common in dark-skinned infants who need greater sun exposure to synthesize adequate amounts of vitamin D. Prolonged breast-feeding increases the risk of rickets as breast milk is a poor source of vitamin D. Infant formulas are often supplemented with vitamin D, but cow's milk is also a poor source of vitamin D. Diseases that interfere with the metabolic conversion and activation of vitamin D, such as severe renal and liver disease, can lead to rickets. Illnesses associated with malabsorption, such as coeliac disease, can also lead to rickets. Other diseases that interfere with calcium and phosphorus homeostasis can cause rickets, e.g. renal tubular defects, such as hypophosphataemic rickets, in which there is failure of phosphate absorption, or Fanconi's syndrome in which there is a defect in the reabsorption of phosphate, glucose and amino acids.

Clinical features include swollen wrists and ankles, frontal bossing, prominent costochondral junctions (a rickety rosary), bow legs or knock-knees, craniotabes, muscle weakness, tetany and hypocalcaemic fits.

The radiograph demonstrates the typical appearance in rickets with widening of the growth plate and cupping, splaying and fraying of the metaphysis.

A vitamin D level to confirm the nutritional aetiology of the rickets and anti-transglutaminase antibody levels to rule out coeliac disease would be helpful.

Iron deficiency anaemia is said to occur in a quarter of children under 5 years of age. Cow's milk is a poor source of iron. Although usually nutritional, blood loss should be considered as a possible cause, especially in older children. This may be due to occult gastrointestinal blood loss secondary to a peptic ulcer, a Meckel's diverticulum or inflammatory bowel disease. A ferritin level should be done to confirm the diagnosis and is likely to be very low. A haemoglobinopathy screen should be performed in high-risk groups to exclude disorders such as thalassaemia that can cause a microcytic hypochromic anaemia and that may coexist with iron deficiency. Infants may be pale, tired, irritable and anorexic. In severe cases they can be tachypnoeic. There is evidence that iron deficiency anaemia can also have adverse effects on attention span and learning.

Treatment consists of a 3-month course of high-dose oral vitamin D. Bone chemistry should be measured 2 weeks after starting treatment and regularly thereafter to avoid hypercalcaemia and to ensure that the biochemical and haematological parameters normalize. This should be followed by maintenance doses of vitamin D for the long term. The prognosis for complete resolution of the deformities is good. In cases where the serum calcium is low, calcium is also given initially until levels normalize.

There is often an accompanying iron deficiency anaemia, as in this case. Red meat and green vegetables are good sources of iron and some foods, such as cereals, are often fortified with iron. The anaemia should be treated with a 3-month course of oral iron.

A dietetic referral and screening of the siblings for rickets and iron deficiency would also be advisable.

 KEY POINTS

- Rickets is usually secondary to inadequate exposure to sunlight and poor nutrition.
- Swollen wrists, a rickety rosary and bow legs are typical clinical features.
- Treatment is with vitamin D.
- Iron deficiency is very common in young children and can be successfully treated with dietary advice and oral iron.

GASTROENTEROLOGY

CASE 23: A VOMITING INFANT

History

Tom is a 7-week-old infant who presents to the A&E department with a 1-week history of non-bilious vomiting. His mother describes the vomit as 'shooting out'. He has a good appetite but has lost 300 g since he was last weighed a week earlier. He has mild constipation. The family have recently returned from Spain. There is no vomiting in any other members of the family. His sister suffers from vesicoureteric reflux and urinary tract infections.

Examination

Tom is apyrexial and mildly dehydrated. His pulse is 170 beats/min, blood pressure 82/43 mmHg, and peripheral capillary refill 2 s. There is no organomegaly, masses or tenderness on abdominal examination. There are no signs in the other systems.

INVESTIGATIONS		
		Normal
Haemoglobin	11.7 g/dL	10.5–13.5 g/dL
White cell count	10.0×10^9/L	$4.0–11.0 \times 10^9$/L
Platelets	332×10^9/L	$150–400 \times 10^9$/L
Sodium	134 mmol/L	135–145 mmol/L
Potassium	3.1 mmol/L	3.5–5.0 mmol/L
Chloride	81 mmol/L	98–106 mmol/L
Urea	9.0 mmol/L	1.8–6.4 mmol/L
Creatinine	60 μmol/L	18–35 μmol/L
Capillary gas		
pH	7.56	7.36–7.44
P_{CO_2}	6.0 kPa	4.0–6.5 kPa
P_{O_2}	3.2 kPa	12–15 kPa
HCO3	38 mmol/L	22–29 mmol/L
Base excess	+10	(−2.5)–(+2.5) mmol/L
Urine dipstick	No abnormality detected	

Questions
- What is the likely diagnosis?
- What is the differential diagnosis?
- How would you confirm the diagnosis?
- What is the treatment?

ANSWER 23

In an infant this age with non-bilious projectile vomiting, pyloric stenosis is the most likely diagnosis. This condition presents between 2 weeks and 5 months of age (median 6 weeks) and projectile vomiting is typical. The vomitus is never bile-stained as the obstruction is proximal to the duodenum. As in this case, infants may also be constipated. The hypochloraemic alkalosis is characteristic and is due to vomiting HCl. The low potassium is due to the kidneys retaining hydrogen ions in favour of potassium ions. The raised urea and creatinine suggest that there is also mild dehydration. The male-to-female ratio is 4:1 and occasionally there is a family history (multifactorial inheritance).

 Differential diagnosis

- Gastro-oesophageal reflux
- Gastritis
- Urinary tract infection
- Overfeeding

Gastro-oesophageal reflux usually presents from or shortly after birth. Gastritis usually occurs with an enteritis and diarrhoea. A urinary infection at this age may present in a very non-specific way and therefore it is mandatory to test the urine. The absence of nitrites and leucocytes in the urine dipstick makes a urinary infection very unlikely. Overfeeding should be elucidated from a careful history.

The diagnosis could be clinically confirmed by carrying out a test feed. A feed leads to peristalsis which occurs from left to right. The abdominal wall is usually relaxed during a feed, making palpation easier. A pyloric mass, which is the size of a 2-cm olive, may be felt in the right hypochodrium by careful palpation. An ultrasound is also usually done for further confirmation.

Tom is slightly tachycardic (pulse rate <1 year, 110–160 beats/min) with a normal blood pressure and capillary refill time. His urea is slightly elevated. Initial treatment consists of treating the dehydration, acid–base and electrolyte abnormalities with intravenous fluids (0.9 per cent saline with 5 per cent dextrose and added KCl would be the appropriate starting fluid in this infant with a low sodium and potassium). Feeds should be stopped, a nasogastric tube inserted and the stomach emptied. The definitive operation is Ramstedt's pyloromyotomy.

KEY POINTS

- The peak age of presentation of pyloric stenosis is 6 weeks.
- The typical biochemical picture is a hypochloraemic alkalosis.
- The definitive treatment is Ramstedt's pyloromyotomy.

CASE 24: A CHILD WITH BLOODY DIARRHOEA

History

Bobby is a 7-month-old child who is referred to the paediatric rapid referral clinic with a 2-day history of diarrhoea with blood and mucus in the stool. His mother states that he has periods of inconsolable crying which are getting worse and more frequent. In the last few hours, he had started to vomit and the last vomit was bile-stained. There is no history of contact with gastroenteritis, of travel or of bleeding disorders. He had neonatal meningitis and subsequently developed epilepsy, which is treated with sodium valproate. He has had no fits in the past month. His mother is in good health but his father has type 1 diabetes.

Examination

He has a temperature of 37.9°C. His pulse rate is 186 beats/min, blood pressure is 80/44 mmHg and capillary refill is 4 s. He is difficult to examine due to frequent crying, but when examined during a quiet period, a mass is felt on the right side of the abdomen. The anus appears normal and there are no other signs.

INVESTIGATIONS		
		Normal
Haemoglobin	12.8 g/dL	10.5–13.5 g/dL
White cell count	7.0×10^9/L	$4.0–11.0 \times 10^9$/L
Platelets	457×10^9/L	$150–400 \times 10^9$/L
Sodium	138 mmol/L	135–145 mmol/L
Potassium	3.9 mmol/L	3.5–5.0 mmol/L
Urea	9.5 mmol/L	1.8–6.4 mmol/L
Creatinine	60 μmol/L	20–80 μmol/L
C-reactive protein	12 mg/L	<6 mg/L

Questions
- What is the diagnosis?
- What is the key investigation?
- What is the treatment?

ANSWER 24

The commonest causes of passing blood per rectum are gastroenteritis and an anal fissure. Gastroenteritis is a possibility in this case, but the lack of contact with gastroenteritis and of recent travel makes it somewhat less likely. The normality of the anus makes an anal fissure unlikely. The age of the child, the rectal bleeding and the mass (a late feature of intussusception) make an intussusception the most likely diagnosis.

The typical age in intussusception is 3 months to 3 years. It is due to a part of the bowel telescoping into the adjacent distal bowel. Most intussusceptions are ileocolic. They result in stretching of the mesenteric vasculature that can potentially lead to bowel ischaemia or infarction. For this reason, investigation and treatment need to be instituted urgently. Typically the child has paroxysmal pain during which he or she becomes very pale; stool containing a mixture of blood and mucus (hence the name redcurrant jelly stool); and a sausage-shaped mass (the intussusception itself) in the upper right quadrant of the abdomen. As the disease progresses, bowel obstruction, peritonitis and septicaemia may develop. The diagnostic investigation is an ultrasound.

! **Causes of rectal bleeding**

- Gastroenteritis
- Anal fissure
- Intussusception
- Cow's milk protein allergy
- Meckel's diverticulum
- Inflammatory bowel disease
- Polyp
- Clotting abnormality
- Sexual abuse

This infant has clinical signs (tachycardia and prolonged capillary refill) and biochemical evidence (raised urea) of dehydration, and initial treatment consists of intravenous fluid resuscitation and intravenous antibiotics, such as penicillin, gentamicin and metronidazole. A nasogastric tube should be inserted and the stomach emptied. In the majority of cases, reduction can be achieved by a radiologist with an air enema. The antibiotics are given because of the possibility of sepsis and the small risk of a perforation during the reduction. If this procedure fails, or if the child is unstable or has signs of peritonitis or a perforation, then surgery is indicated. There is a recurrence rate of 10 per cent following an air enema reduction, and of 2–5 per cent following a surgical reduction.

 KEY POINTS

- Intussusception should be considered in any child aged 3 months to 3 years with bloody stool.
- There should be a low threshold for carrying out an ultrasound.
- An air enema reduction is successful in the majority of cases.

CASE 25: A TEENAGER WITH CHRONIC DIARRHOEA

History

Levi is a 14-year-old boy who presents to the paediatric rapid referral clinic with a 3-week history of diarrhoea and cramp-like abdominal pain. He has no blood or mucus in his stool and has had no vomiting. His appetite is poor and he has lost 3.5 kg in 3 weeks. He has intermittent fevers. The family recently returned from France where his father contracted diarrhoea, from which he is now recovering. There is no other medical history of note. His mother suffers from irritable bowel syndrome.

Examination

He looks generally unwell. There is no anaemia, jaundice, clubbing or lymphadenopathy. His temperature is 37.9°C. There is generalized abdominal tenderness but no guarding or rebound. There is no organomegaly. Inspection of the mouth and anus is normal. His pubertal assessment shows him to have testes that are 5 mL in volume and pubic hair and genitalia that are Tanner stage 2.

His weight, at 35 kg, is on the second centile and his height, at 151 cm, is on the ninth centile (mid-parental height is on the 50th centile).

INVESTIGATIONS		
		Normal
Haemoglobin	10.9 g/dL	14–18 g/dL
White cell count	15.2×10^9/L	$4.0–11.0 \times 10^9$/L
Platelets	623×10^9/L	$150–400 \times 10^9$/L
Mean cell volume	70 fL	76–96 fL
Erythrocyte sedimentation rate (ESR)	87 mm/h	<15 mm/h
C-reactive protein (CRP)	36 mg/L	<6 mg/L
Ferritin	14 ng/ml	20–300 ng/ml
Albumin	31 g/L	35–50 g/L
Urea and electrolytes	Normal	
Stool – no bacterial growth, no ova, cysts or parasites		

Questions
- What is the most likely diagnosis?
- What investigations would you do?
- What is the initial treatment?

ANSWER 25

The most likely diagnosis is Crohn's disease. The most important differentials are an infective enteropathy (e.g. *Campylobacter*, *Yersinia*, *Giardia*) and ulcerative colitis. Tenderness may be over the terminal ileum in the right iliac fossa, but can also be generalized, and signs may mimic those of an acute abdomen. The father's resolving diarrhoea is most likely to be coincidental. The irritable bowel syndrome does not lead to weight loss, fevers and abnormal blood results, as in this case. It is very important to examine the anus in cases of suspected Crohn's, as perianal disease (e.g. skin tags, abscess, fistula) is present in 45 per cent of patients. Clubbing may also be present. This child has a degree of growth failure and delayed puberty, which is common in adolescents with Crohn's disease. The microcytic anaemia in Crohn's is due to a combination of gastrointestinal blood loss, an insufficient dietary intake and inadequate iron absorption. The white cell count and platelets are often raised. The ESR and CRP are usually elevated and the albumin is often low due to malabsorption and protein loss in the stool. The most common extraintestinal manifestation (10 per cent) is arthritis, typically affecting large joints. The most common dermatological manifestations are erythema nodosum and pyoderma gangrenosum. All patients require an expert ophthalmic examination, which may reveal episcleritis or uveitis.

! Causes of chronic diarrhoea (>14 days)

Infection
- Bacterial (*Salmonella*, *Campylobacter*)
- Protozoal (e.g. *Giardia*)
- Post-gastroenteritis diarrhoea

Malabsorption
- Lactose intolerance
- Cow's milk protein intolerance
- Cystic fibrosis
- Coeliac disease

Gastrointestinal disorders
- Crohn's disease
- Ulcerative colitis

Miscellaneous
- Toddler's diarrhoea/irritable bowel syndrome
- Drugs (e.g. laxatives, antibiotics, chemotherapy)
- Immunodeficiency

A colonoscopy with colonic and terminal ileal biopsies should be performed. An upper gastrointestinal endoscopy should also be done in all new cases of suspected Crohn's disease, as clinically significant upper tract disease can be present in the absence of upper gastrointestinal symptoms.

The goals of treatment are to achieve clinical remission and to promote growth with adequate nutrition. Patients with mild disease are treated with preparations of 5-aminosalicylic acid, e.g. sulphasalazine, antibiotics such as metronidazole and nutritional therapy.

If there is no response, corticosteroids and immunosuppressive therapy with 6-mercaptopurine or methotrexate can be tried. The latter two agents can also have corticosteroid-sparing effects. Surgery is considered when medical therapy fails. Indications include intractable disease with growth failure, obstruction (due to strictures or adhesions), abscess drainage, fistula, intractable haemorrhage and perforation.

 KEY POINTS

- The perianal area should always be examined in cases of suspected Crohn's disease.
- Growth failure and delayed puberty are common in Crohn's disease.
- Colonoscopy and upper gastrointestinal endoscopy are key investigations.
- Initial treatment consists of preparations of 5-aminosalicylic acid, antibiotics and nutritional therapy.

CASE 26: ACUTE DIARRHOEA AND VOMITING

History

Luca is a 24-month-old boy with Down's syndrome, brought to the A&E department by his mother. He has had diarrhoea and vomiting for 1 day. In the last 8 hours, he has drunk 200 ml milk, vomited five times and passed six liquid stools. The vomit is not bilious and there is no blood or mucus in the stools. It has been hard to tell if he is passing urine because every nappy is soiled. He has no cardiac problems and no other medical problems except glue ear. There is no history of foreign travel. His two older siblings have recently had diarrhoea and vomiting.

Examination

He is miserable and lethargic. His heart rate is 120 beats/min, respiratory rate is 25 breaths/min, and his temperature is 37.7°C. He has dry mucous membranes, his eyes are slightly sunken, his skin turgor appears normal and his capillary refill time is less than 2 s. His abdomen is soft with no masses palpable. His weight is 11 kg (50th centile on the Down's syndrome growth chart).

An oral fluid challenge is commenced in the emergency department. He drinks 60 ml of electrolyte solution over 2 hours and vomits once on the floor. He does not pass urine into a urine bag during this period.

Questions

- What is the most likely diagnosis?
- How dehydrated is this child?
- How would you manage this child now?
- How would you calculate the fluid requirements for this child over the next 24 hours?

ANSWERS 26

The most likely diagnosis is viral gastroenteritis, probably due to rotavirus. This fits with the acute onset and the fact that his siblings have also been unwell.

This child is about 5 per cent dehydrated, which means that he has lost 5 per cent of his body weight as fluid. Signs of dehydration in children are shown in Table 26.1.

Table 26.1 Signs of dehydration in children

	Mild (<5 per cent)	Moderate (5–10 per cent)	Severe (>10 per cent)
Oral mucosa	Dry	Dry	Dry
Eyes	Normal	Sunken	Very sunken
Fontanelle	Normal	Sunken	Very sunken
Skin turgor	Normal	Reduced	Very reduced
Pulse	Normal	Fast	Fast and weak
Capillary refill time	Normal	Prolonged	Prolonged
Blood pressure	Normal	Normal	Low
Urine output	Normal	Reduced	Very reduced
Mental state	Normal	Lethargic	Irritable or obtunded

Management of mild-to-moderate dehydration should involve enteral rehydration (oral or nasogastric) whenever possible. This can be done with an appropriate electrolyte solution. After an initial 4-hour period of rehydration (when the fluid deficit is replaced), normal feeds can be resumed, although breast-feeding can be continued throughout. Intravenous rehydration is associated with a slower recovery and a longer hospital stay but is necessary if a child needs acute volume replacement for shock or is unable to tolerate enteral fluids. Luca should be admitted for a trial of nasogastric fluid therapy. If he does not tolerate this, he will probably need intravenous rehydration. This is calculated as follows:

Fluid requirement for 24 hours = maintenance + correction of deficit + replacement of ongoing losses

Maintenance fluid = 100 mL/kg for first 10 kg body weight = 100 × 10
           + 50 mL/kg for next 10 kg   = 50 × 1
           + 20 mL/kg thereafter
                                 Total = 1050

His fluid deficit is 5 per cent of body weight = (5/100) × 11 kg = 0.55 kg. This is equivalent to 550 mL (1 mL of water weighs 1 g). Losses (stool and vomit) are calculated from the fluid balance chart and can be replaced at regular intervals. For this child, the total fluid requirement for the first 24 hours is calculated as follows:

1050 mL + 550 mL + losses = 1600 mL + losses

This is equivalent to 67 mL/hour + losses.

🔑 | **KEY POINTS**

- Rotavirus is the most common cause of gastroenteritis in infants and young children.
- Clinical assessment of dehydration is based on multiple physical signs.
- Where possible, enteral rehydration with an electrolyte solution should be used for children with gastroenteritis.
- Fluid replacement must account for the deficit plus the maintenance requirement plus ongoing losses.

History

Sarah is a 13-year-old girl who is brought to the A&E department by her mother, with a 2-day history of abdominal pain and vomiting. She got back from a family holiday in Devon yesterday evening and has been feeling unwell since. Initially she had central abdominal pain which was coming and going, but now she has more constant pain on the right side of her abdomen. She has vomited three times, but her stool has been normal. She has no significant medical history, was well during the 2 weeks in Devon and her last period was about 2 weeks ago. Her family are all well and report that they all ate the same food over the last few weeks.

Examination

She is flushed and has a temperature of 37.9°C. Her heart rate is 95 beats/min, respiratory rate is 18 breaths/min, capillary refill time is less than 2s, and blood pressure is 105/67 mmHg. She appears obese (weight 68 kg, 98th centile; height 151 cm, 25th centile). Her abdomen is tender in the right lower quadrant but there is no guarding or rebound tenderness. Pressing in the left lower quadrant elicits pain on the right.

INVESTIGATIONS		
		Normal
Haemoglobin	12.3 g/dL	12.1–15.1 g/dL
White cell count	16.3 × 10⁹/L	4.5–13 × 10⁹/L
Neutrophil count	10 × 10⁹/L	1.5–6 × 10⁹/L
Platelets	210 × 10⁹/L	180–430 × 10⁹/L
Sodium	133 mmol/L	135–145 mmol/L
Potassium	3.4 mmol/L	3.5–5.6 mmol/L
Urea	4.3 mmol/L	2.5–6.6 mmol/L
Creatinine	76 μmol/L	20–80 μmol/L
Bilirubin	5 mmol/L	1.7–26 mmol/L
Alkaline phosphatase	264 IU/dL	25–800 IU/dL
Aspartate aminotransferase	20 IU/dL	10–45 IU/dL
Albumin	35 g/L	37–50 g/L
C-reactive protein	16 mg/L	<5 mg/L
Urine		
Leucocytes	+	Negative
Nitrites	Negative	Negative
Blood	Negative	Negative

Ultrasound abdomen – liver, spleen and kidneys appear normal. There are a few slightly enlarged mesenteric lymph nodes. The appendix is not seen.

Questions
- What is the most likely diagnosis?
- What other diagnoses should be considered?
- How should she be managed?

ANSWER 27

The most likely diagnosis is appendicitis. This is consistent with the history, the signs on examination, the low-grade fever, raised white cell count and neutrophilia. Vomiting, and even diarrhoea can be features of appendicitis and do not always indicate gastro-enteritis. Sterile pyuria (leucocytes in the urine, without organisms) can be caused by the inflamed appendix irritating the ureter or bladder.

Plain radiographs are usually normal unless there has been perforation of the appendix. Ultrasound can confirm the diagnosis of appendicitis but can miss an inflamed appen-dix, particularly if the subject is obese or the appendix is retrocaecal. CT scanning has better sensitivity and specificity but involves a high radiation dose. There is no perfect test for appendicitis, and in practice it remains a clinical diagnosis. If there is diag-nostic uncertainty, repeated clinical examination and ultrasound are often performed. When the diagnosis is clear clinically, substantially delaying surgery to allow imaging can result in perforation of the appendix.

! Causes of right lower quadrant pain
<ul><li>Appendicitis</li><li>Mesenteric adenitis</li><li>Urinary tract infection</li><li>Gastroenteritis</li><li>Crohn's disease</li><li>Ovulation pain: 'mittelschmerz'</li><li>Ovarian cyst/torsion</li><li>Ectopic pregnancy</li><li>Pelvic inflammatory disease</li></ul>

Sarah should be admitted to hospital for a surgical opinion. She should have nil by mouth until the decision is made on whether or not to operate. Unfortunately, her abdominal pain was unconvincing when she was seen by the surgical team and so she was admitted for observation with a plan to repeat the ultrasound the next day. She developed worsen-ing abdominal pain and peritonism the next morning and was taken to theatre, where a perforated appendix was removed and she had a 10-day in-patient stay complicated by sepsis and ileus.

KEY POINTS
<ul><li>The triad of abdominal pain, vomiting and a low-grade fever is suggestive of appendicitis.</li><li>The diagnosis is primarily clinical as there is no perfect test to rule in or rule out appendicitis.</li><li>A prompt diagnosis is important to avoid perforation and peritonitis.</li></ul>

History

Danielle is an 8-year-girl referred to children's outpatients by her GP. She has been seen several times by different partners over the previous couple of years with abdominal pain. She describes the pain as peri-umbilical, non-radiating, sometimes sharp, but usually an ache. There is no obvious periodicity, including to food. Her appetite is good and there are no concerns about her growth and weight gain. She has her bowels open most days and there has never been any blood or mucus. She occasionally feels nauseated with the pain but has never vomited. There are no urinary symptoms. She started junior school last year and moved house around the same time after her parents separated. She lives with her mother, but she and her 4-year-old brother have frequent contact with their father. She was doing well at infants but is now falling behind, having missed quite a lot of school. She has several badges for gymnastics. There is no family history of note, including migraine. Her mother is worried that this is something to do with puberty and that her periods are about to start.

Examination

Danielle is a generally healthy, cooperative, but slightly anxious girl. Her nails are bitten but there is no clubbing, anaemia, lymphadenopathy or jaundice. Her height is on the 25th centile and her weight is on the 9th. She is prepubertal. Full examination is normal.

INVESTIGATIONS		
		Normal
Haemoglobin	12.3 g/dL	11.5–15.5 g/dL
White cell count	8.4×10^9/L	$6-17.5 \times 10^9$/L
Platelets	365×10^9/L	$150-400 \times 10^9$/L
Sodium	138 mmol/L	138–146 mmol/L
Potassium	4.5 mmol/L	3.5–5.0 mmol/L
Urea	4.2 mmol/L	1.8–6.4 mmol/L
Creatinine	46 μmol/L	27–62 μmol/L
C-reactive protein	<6 mg/L	<6 mg/L
Immunoglobulins	Normal	
Transglutaminase antibodies	Negative	
Midstream urine	Normal	
Abdominal ultrasound	Normal	

Questions

- What is the most likely diagnosis?
- What is the differential diagnosis?
- How would you manage this patient?

ANSWER 28

The most likely diagnosis is chronic abdominal pain of childhood or recurrent abdominal pain (RAP). This is a benign, very common but potentially debilitating condition. The pointers to this not being organic are the chronicity of the characteristic symptoms in an otherwise healthy, physically active child. The commonest identifiable cause for RAP is psychosomatic, as seems likely from the description of this girl who has had many recent changes in her life. However, it is a diagnosis of exclusion and investigations exclude conditions that can have an insidious onset, such as coeliac disease, and reassure the child and family that there is no sinister cause. The latter is crucial because the symptoms are very real and there is understandable anxiety.

Among the differentials, abdominal migraine differs in that it is usually associated with pallor and vomiting. There is almost always a family history of migraine. An organic cause is also more likely the further the pain is from the umbilicus.

Mothers often worry that RAP heralds menarche but this comes towards the end of puberty. Sexual abuse should be considered in the differential.

!   **Differential diagnosis of chronic abdominal pain**
• Psychosomatic
• Urinary tract infections
• Constipation
• Gastro-oesophageal reflux
• Coeliac disease
• Inflammatory bowel disease
• Cow's milk intolerance
• Abnormal renal anatomy, e.g. pelviureteric junction obstruction
• Abdominal migraine
• Peptic ulcer
• Sexual or other abuse

Management focuses on explanations and reassurance. It is helpful to liken the condition to tension headaches in adults – common and unpleasant but not serious. Acknowledge that there is no question of fabrication. Children rarely fabricate symptoms and, if they do, abuse should be considered. The classic time for RAP is in the morning before school. Most parents recognize this and have often already asked questions about bullying or other worries, but sometimes a cycle sets in where missing school and falling behind worsen the symptoms and cause more anxiety. The child may be recognized as a 'worrier' and most can understand the concept of psychosomatic symptoms.

Some families still find it difficult to accept that there is nothing medically wrong and pursue a diagnosis such as food allergy. They may seek advice from practitioners of alternative medicine and it is important to discuss openly the dangers of dietary exclusions that they may suggest. In the absence of other symptoms, such as diarrhoea or an association with eating, there is no evidence that such measures are effective.

Once a diagnosis has been reached, the child should be discharged from hospital follow-up to prevent the risk of reinforcing a medical diagnosis. Referral to a psychologist or psychiatrist is sometimes necessary.

KEY POINTS

- Children can have psychosomatic symptoms just as adults – however, these are a diagnosis of exclusion.

CASE 29: A CONSTIPATED TODDLER

History

Tanya is a 4-year-old girl who presents to outpatients with a 2-year history of constipation. She opens her bowels about once every 5 days and strains. She soils her knickers on most days. She has intermittent abdominal pain, which is relieved by opening her bowels. Recently, there has been fresh blood on the toilet tissue. Lactulose has been used, with little success. Her mother states that she did not have a dirty nappy until 40 hours of age.

She has recently had a urine infection diagnosed by her GP. The illness was mild and responded well to antibiotics. She was delivered by emergency Caesarean section because of fetal distress and meconium staining.

Examination

A faecal mass is palpable in the left iliac fossa. The anus appears normal. Rectal examination – hard stool palpated. The back is normal. Blood pressure is 101/62 mmHg. There are no other signs. Weight is on the 50th centile and height is on the 25th centile.

Questions
- What is the most likely diagnosis?
- Would you carry out any investigations?
- What is the treatment?

ANSWER 29

The most likely diagnosis is functional constipation. This condition is associated with faecal masses in the lower abdomen. Severe constipation can lead to an anal fissure (and vice versa). This is the likely cause of the bleeding. It may be high up in the anus and therefore not visible on inspection. The soiling is involuntary and due to liquid stool leaking from above the hard stool mass in the rectum. Hirschsprung's disease should be suspected if meconium has not been passed in the first 24 hours of life. However, in this case, the passage of meconium *in utero*, the lack of symptoms in the first 2 years of life and the normal weight make that diagnosis unlikely. Furthermore, in Hirschsprung's disease the rectum is usually empty.

! **Causes of constipation**

- Dietary
- Dehydration
- Anal fissure/stenosis
- Hirschsprung's disease
- Intestinal obstruction e.g. stricture post-necrotizing enterocolitis
- Spinal cord lesion
- Cystic fibrosis (meconium ileus equivalent)
- Cow's milk intolerance
- Drugs, e.g. opiates, vincristine, lead poisoning
- Hypothyroidism
- Sexual abuse

No investigations are necessary. Usually, clinical assessment suffices to make the diagnosis. In children who refuse a rectal examination, or if there is doubt about the diagnosis, then an abdominal X-ray is useful to assess the degree of faecal loading. Children with constipation are more likely to get urinary infections. In a 4-year-old with a history of one, non-severe urinary tract infection, no investigations are required.

Dietary advice needs to be given, encouraging a good fluid intake, a daily high-fibre cereal and fruit and vegetables. Star charts may also help.

Initial drug treatment consists of an osmotic laxative such as lactulose. If that is ineffective, as in this case, a stimulant laxative such as senna should be added. If the patient remains constipated, a more powerful osmotic laxative such as Movicol can be used as a single agent. The doses of these medications can be titrated to the frequency of bowel actions, with the aim being for the child to open their bowels daily in a pain-free manner without soiling.

If the child has pain secondary to an anal fissure, lidocaine ointment should help. Whenever possible, treatment is administered orally. However, in some cases glycerine suppositories or phosphate enemas are required to help disimpact hard stool in the rectum.

In very severe cases, a bowel-cleansing solution such as Klean-Prep may be needed, and in extreme cases a manual evacuation may need to be performed in theatre.

Constipation often starts at the age of 2 years when the child is being toilet-trained. Toilet training may lead to 'power struggles' between the child and the family and thus to constipation. In some cases, psychological intervention is helpful.

KEY POINTS

- Functional constipation is very common.
- Investigations are usually unnecessary.
- Initial treatment consists of dietary advice and lactulose.

CASE 30: AN INFANT WITH POOR WEIGHT GAIN

History

Tommy is a 9-month-old boy who is referred to the outpatient clinic with failure to thrive. His birth weight was 3.17 kg, he gained weight well initially and was weaned at 6 months. His appetite has been poor over the last couple of months and his mother describes him as miserable. He has no vomiting and opens his bowels four times a day. The stool is loose and smelly but contains no blood or mucus. His mother breast-fed until 4 months of age. The family have recently returned from Turkey but his mother states that the poor feeding and weight loss preceded their holiday. His father has Crohn's disease, for which he has required several operations.

Examination

Tommy is a thin, pale-looking infant. He is miserable and cries easily, and his abdomen is distended. There are no signs of tenderness, masses or organomegaly. The oral cavity and perianal area appear normal. There are no other signs. His centile chart is in Figure 30.1.

INVESTIGATIONS		
		Normal
Haemoglobin	8.2 g/dL	9.0–14.0 g/dL
Mean cell volume	68 fL	70–86 fL
White cell count	9.8×10^9/L	$4.0–11.0 \times 10^9$/L
Platelets	432×10^9/L	$150–400 \times 10^9$/L
C-reactive protein	9 mg/L	< 6 mg/L
Ferritin	6 ng/ml	15–200 ng/ml
Urea and electrolytes	Normal	
Liver function tests	Normal	
Bone chemistry	Normal	
Immunoglobulins	Normal	
Coeliac screen		
Transglutaminase IgA Antibody	>100 U/mL	0–8 U/mL
Urine dip	Negative	
Stool – no bacterial growth, no ova, cysts or parasites		

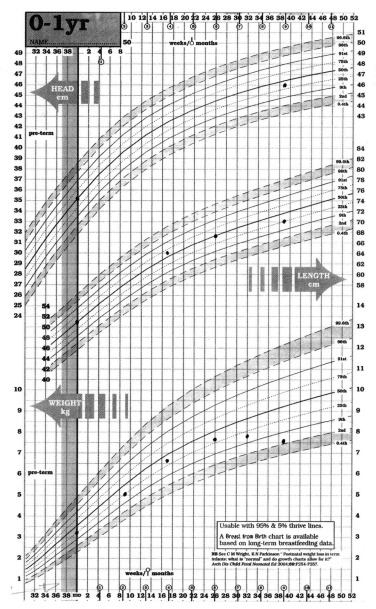

Figure 30.1 Centile chart. (Chart reproduced with kind permission of the Child Growth Foundation.)

Questions
- What is the definition of failure to thrive?
- What are the causes of failure to thrive?
- What is the likely diagnosis and how could it be confirmed?

ANSWER 30

Failure to thrive is a descriptive term and not a diagnosis. It is often defined as a weight, or a rate of weight gain, that is significantly below what is normal for a child of that age and sex. Some authors define failure to thrive as a weight that has fallen two centile lines on the standard growth charts. Although this term can refer to height as well as weight, it is usually used in relation to weight in children under 2 years of age.

! Causes of failure to thrive

Inadequate intake of food
- Poor feeding
- Mechanical problem such as a cleft palate or bulbar palsy

Malabsorption
- Coeliac disease
- Cystic fibrosis

Excessive loss of nutrients
- Vomiting due to gastro-oesophageal reflux
- Protein-losing enteropathy, e.g. cow's milk protein intolerance

Increased nutrient requirement
- Congestive cardiac failure
- Chronic infection, e.g. HIV

Miscellaneous causes
- Dysmorphic syndromes, e.g. Russell–Silver syndrome
- Inborn errors of metabolism

Psychosocial
- Child abuse and neglect
- Emotional and social deprivation

It is important to take a full dietary history. The commonest cause of failure to thrive is a poor nutrient intake which may be due to feeding mismanagement or psychosocial problems. Failure to thrive may also be the result of a combination of the factors in the above box, and in some cases no cause is found. Crohn's disease is very rare in this age group and the father's illness is coincidental.

The likely diagnosis is coeliac disease. Steatorrhoea (with pale, greasy, smelly stool) and diarrhoea are typical. The abdominal distension is due to distension of the intestinal loops with fluids and gas. The centile chart shows that the weight has crossed two centile lines since 6 months and that there has also been weight loss. This would correspond with weaning at 6 months and the introduction of gluten in wheat and other foods. The anaemia is secondary to the poor nutrient intake and malabsorption. Folate as well as iron deficiency may occur. Anti-tissue transglutaminase is >95 per cent accurate in diagnosing coeliac disease (it is important to simultaneously measure IgA, as anti-tissue transglutaminase is an IgA antibody and IgA deficiency would invalidate the test). However, the definitive diagnosis is based on an endoscopy with a jejunal biopsy. In cases of coeliac disease, there is subtotal villous atrophy, crypt hypertrophy and a lamina propria plasma cell infiltrate. Treatment is with a gluten-free diet.

KEY POINTS

- The commonest cause of failure to thrive is a poor nutrient intake.
- Serological testing is very useful in the diagnosis of coeliac disease, but definitive diagnosis is with a jejunal biopsy.
- Treatment of coeliac disease is with a gluten-free diet.

CASE 31: AN INFANT WITH PERSISTENT JAUNDICE

History

Matthew is referred by the community midwife because he is still jaundiced at 3 weeks of age. He is seen in the paediatric clinic at 4 weeks of age. He was born at 39 weeks' gestation by ventouse delivery and is the first child. His birth weight was 3.8 kg (75th centile). His mother had gestational diabetes controlled by diet alone. All antenatal scans and screening blood tests were normal. His mother's blood group is O-positive. He has been well since birth.

Examination

Matthew's weight is 4.5 kg (50th centile). On examination, his face, trunk and upper limbs are jaundiced. He is not dysmorphic, he has no bruising, and cardiovascular and respiratory examinations are normal. Abdominal examination reveals a firm liver edge 4 cm below the costal margin and a small umbilical granuloma.

INVESTIGATIONS		
		Normal
Urinalysis		
Urobilinogen	Negative	Positive
Bilirubin	++	Negative
Reducing substances	Negative	Negative
Blood		
Haemoglobin	13.4 g/dL	10.7–17.1 g/dL
White cell count	8×10^9/L	$6–21 \times 10^9$/L
Platelets	205×10^9/L	$17–500 \times 10^9$/L
Reticulocytes	30×10^9/L	$10–80 \times 10^9$/L
Blood group	O Rhesus positive	
Thyroid-stimulating hormone	4.6 mU/L	0.3–5.0 mU/L
Free thyroxine	13 pmol/L	9–23 pmol/L
Total bilirubin	140 mmol/L	1.7–26 mmol/L (after 1 month)
Conjugated bilirubin	110 mmol/L	<15 per cent of total

Questions
- What additional questions should be asked to help determine the diagnosis?
- What is the likely cause of this infant's prolonged jaundice?
- How would you manage this baby?

ANSWER 31

The history should establish when jaundice first occurred, as the causes of early-onset jaundice are different from the causes of prolonged jaundice. Parents should be asked specifically about the presence of pale stools and dark urine. Pale stool indicates that bile pigments are not being excreted into the gut, and dark urine occurs with the accumulation of water-soluble conjugated bilirubin in the urine. These indicate that there is obstruction to bile flow out of the liver. The urine dipstick shows the presence of bilirubin but the absence of urobilinogen, so this child would be expected to have pale stools and dark urine.

! **Neonatal jaundice requiring investigation**

- Early onset, <24–36 hours after birth
- Severe jaundice, at any time (definition of severe jaundice varies with age)
- Prolonged, >14 days

The causes of neonatal jaundice, including prolonged jaundice, are outlined in Case 82 (p. 243).

Prolonged conjugated hyperbilirubinaemia in a baby who appears well is likely to be due to extrahepatic biliary atresia. Progressive destruction of the extrahepatic bile ducts occurs, with obstruction of bile flow and, subsequently, rapid progression of damage within the liver and cirrhosis.

It is important to pick up cases of extrahepatic biliary atresia early, so that the diagnosis can be confirmed by ultrasound and liver biopsy and then surgery can be performed before irreversible damage to the liver has occurred. The outcome of the Kasai procedure (portoenterostomy) is much better for surgery performed before 60 days of age. For this reason, the case needs to be discussed promptly with the local specialist centre.

 KEY POINTS

- In prolonged neonatal jaundice with a raised conjugated bilirubin fraction, the diagnosis must be extrahepatic biliary atresia until proven otherwise.
- The outcome of the Kasai procedure is much better if surgery is performed early.

History

Ferdinand is a 12-year-old boy who is brought to the A&E department by his parents. This is his third attendance in the last 2 weeks. Today he has been complaining of abdominal pain and his parents noticed that the whites of his eyes look yellow. He has been scratching himself a lot, although he has not had a rash. The notes from his previous attendances show that he had a flu-like illness with a fever up to 38.5°C, nausea and a poor appetite over the last 10 days. However, there were no abnormal findings on examination. He has previously been healthy, but he did travel to the Philippines in the school holidays about 5 weeks ago. He was born in the UK and received all his routine childhood immunizations.

Examination

He is jaundiced and appears in discomfort. His temperature is 36.8°C, heart rate is 90 beats/min, respiratory rate 20/min, oxygen saturation 98 per cent in air, and his blood pressure is 118/70 mmHg. Cardiovascular and respiratory examinations are normal, but his liver is palpable 4 cm below the costal margin and is tender. Ears, nose and throat are normal and he is alert and fully orientated.

INVESTIGATIONS		
		Normal
Haemoglobin	12.3 g/dL	12.1–16.6 g/dL
White cell count	11.9 × 10⁹/L	4.5–13 × 10⁹/L
Platelets	250 × 10⁹/L	180–430 × 10⁹/L
Bilirubin	89 mmol/L	1.7–26 mmol/L
Alkaline phosphatase	1050	25–800 IU/dL
Aspartate aminotransferase	3798	10–45 IU/dL
Albumin	35	37–50 g/L

Questions

- What other questions are important to ask the patient and family?
- What additional tests would be useful?
- What is the most likely diagnosis?
- How could this illness have been prevented?

ANSWER 32

The history can be very helpful in establishing whether jaundice is caused by a pre-hepatic, hepatic or posthepatic problem. Bilirubin is produced by degradation of haem and is initially unconjugated, and hence water-insoluble. Unconjugated bilirubin is transported bound to albumin and is conjugated in the liver parenchymal cells to make it water-soluble and excretable in bile. Conjugated bilirubin is excreted and converted to urobilinogen, urobilin and stercobilinogen in the gut, which can be reabsorbed, leading to the enterohepatic circulation of bile pigments. These pigments give stool its normal coloration. If there is increased unconjugated bilirubin production from increased red cell destruction (e.g. haemolysis) then there will be jaundice with normally pigmented stool and urine. If there is obstruction to bile excretion (e.g. common bile duct stone), conjugated bilirubin accumulates (which causes itching), overflows into urine (causing it to appear dark), and does not reach the gut (resulting in pale stools). Hepatic causes may produce a combination of these patterns. Thus it is important to ask about stool and urine colour, as well as factors that may predispose to each type of cause. In this case, a full travel history is necessary and additional questions should be asked about pre-travel immunization and drug history.

! **Differential diagnosis of abdominal pain and jaundice**

Pre-hepatic
- Abdominal pain is an uncommon feature
- Possible causes: malaria, sickle cell crisis

Hepatic
- Often pale stools and dark urine will be present
- Acute hepatitis due to infection, drugs, toxins

Posthepatic
- Pale stools and dark urine
- Bile duct stones, cholecystitis, choledochal cyst
- Cholangitis must be considered in a febrile child

Additional tests should include urine dipstick to confirm bilirubinuria, amylase, determination of the conjugated and unconjugated fractions of serum bilirubin, serological investigation for viral hepatitis (most importantly, hepatitis A IgM), a clotting profile and abdominal ultrasound.

The most likely diagnosis is hepatitis A, which is uncommon in the UK but endemic throughout much of the world and is most likely to cause symptomatic acute hepatitis in older children and adults. There is usually a flu-like prodromal phase, with nausea and anorexia starting 2–6 weeks after exposure, followed by an icteric phase when there may be tender hepatomegaly. Usually children make a complete recovery. Other infections (e.g. hepatitis B, or C, and Epstein–Barr virus) can also cause acute hepatitis but are less common.

Hepatitis A can be prevented by immunization and good hygiene practices, as it is transmitted by the faeco-oral route.

 KEY POINTS

- Always ask about urine and stool colour in a jaundiced child.
- Hepatitis A is endemic throughout much of the world.
- Hepatitis A is most likely to cause symptomatic disease in older children and adults

---

CASE 33: A LUMP IN THE GROIN

History

William is a 10-month-old boy who presents to his GP with swelling of the left side of his scrotum. His parents first noticed this about 2 weeks previously whilst he was in the bath. By the next morning, it seemed to have disappeared but since then they have noticed it intermittently. It does not seem to be causing him any distress. William was born by emergency Caesarean section at 34 weeks' gestation after serial scans showed poor intrauterine growth. His birth weight was 1.6 kg (2nd centile). The placenta was in poor condition. His neonatal course was uneventful and he is making good developmental progress.

Examination

William's weight is 7.8 kg (9th centile) and his length is 70.5 cm (50th centile), correcting for his prematurity. He is a healthy, cheerful active boy. Initial examination of the genitalia appears normal, with both testes palpable within the scrotum and no asymmetry. However, he then begins to struggle and a smooth firm swelling appears in the left inguinal region and there is distension of the left hemiscrotum. With gentle pressure, it disappears. The remainder of the examination is unremarkable.

Questions
- What is the most likely diagnosis?
- What is the cause in children?
- Which groups of children are most at risk?
- What is the treatment?

ANSWER 33

The site and intermittent nature of the swelling make an inguinal hernia the most likely diagnosis. They are sometimes difficult to detect. Older children can increase their intra-abdominal pressure by coughing, and examining them standing up may help. The position of the testes must be noted because, if retractile, they can be mistaken for a hernia. In girls the contents of the hernial sac are often adherent within the sac and hence not reducible – a sliding hernia – and a fallopian tube or ovary may be palpable. The commonest cause of a swelling in the groin is a lymph node, but they are usually small and mobile and lie more inferior and lateral than an inguinal hernia. They may also be confused with a retractile testis. An ultrasound can help. Direct and femoral hernias are rare in children.

In adults, inguinal hernias are associated with a muscular weakness or defect, but in children they usually result from persistent patency of the processus vaginalis (PV). This accompanies the testis as it exits the abdomen and descends into the scrotum and is obliterated by, or soon after, birth. Failure of obliteration can occur anywhere along its length, explaining the range of presentations (see Fig. 33.1). A hydrocoele is fluid within the tunica vaginalis – the remnant of the PV that surrounds the testis. Hydrocoeles trans-illuminate. They usually resolve spontaneously by the age of 12 months and, if not, should be referred to a surgeon. Fifty per cent of inguinal hernias present in the first year of life, most by the age of 6 months.

! Children at risk of inguinal hernia

- Preterm infants – especially those with very low birth weight (~30 per cent affected)
- Boys – outnumber girls 6:1 because ovaries do not leave the abdominal cavity
- Infants with chronic lung disease
- Children with conditions associated with abnormal abdominal fluid or increased intra-abdominal pressure
- Children with developmental urogenital anomalies
- Infants with disorders of sexual differentiation – phenotypically female infants with inguinal hernias, especially bilateral, should be examined carefully to exclude complete androgen insensitivity syndrome, an extremely rare but crucial diagnosis

---

Treatment is surgical. Early repair reduces the significant risk of the contents of the sac becoming irreducible (incarceration) and/or the hernia becoming strangulated, i.e. so tightly constricted that the contents become ischaemic or gangrenous, with consequent testicular atrophy.

🔑 KEY POINTS

- The commonest cause of a lump in the groin is a lymph node
- Preterm infants are at high risk of developing an inguinal hernia
- Early repair of a hernia is important to reduce the risk of incarceration and/or strangulation

---

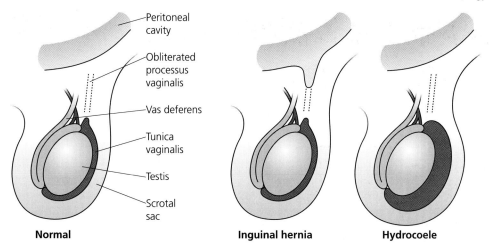

Figure 33.1 Schematic diagram of development of inguinal hernia and hydrocoele.

NEPHROLOGY

CASE 34: ABDOMINAL PAIN AND DYSURIA

History
Leah is a 5-year-old girl who has been passing urine frequently for the last 2 days and complaining of pain when doing so. Her parents have brought her to A&E today because they measured a temperature of 39°C using a forehead thermometer and she had an episode of violent shivering. She has also complained of pain in her back and has vomited three times today.

Leah had oesophageal atresia with a tracheo-oesophageal fistula diagnosed at birth. Her parents remember that some tests were done at birth but no other abnormalities were found. She has no history of urinary infections. They have moved home four times since she was born and have not had any follow-up for years. She is generally healthy and has recently started school, which she enjoys.

Examination
She is flushed and miserable. Her temperature is 39.1°C, heart rate 130 beats/min, respiratory rate 25/min, and her oxygen saturation is 99 per cent in air. Capillary refill is 2 s, heart sounds are normal and her chest is clear. She has a mild kyphoscoliosis. Her abdomen feels soft and is not distended, but there is significant discomfort when palpating the right loin. Her external genitalia appear normal. Her weight is 17 kg (25th centile).

INVESTIGATIONS		
		Normal
Urine dipstick		
Leucocytes	+++	Negative
Nitrites	Positive	Negative
Blood	Trace	Negative
Glucose	Negative	Negative
Protein	Negative	Negative

Questions
- What is the diagnosis?
- How would you manage this child?
- What underlying diagnosis might be considered?

ANSWER 34

This child's clinical features and urine dipstick results are consistent with a urinary tract infection (UTI). The combination of leucocytes and nitrites on urine dipstick is highly predictive of a UTI. Urine dipstick should be a routine part of the assessment of a febrile child. It is important to recognize that the history and physical findings suggest that this is more than just cystitis. She has probably had a rigor, which may indicate bacterial products entering the bloodstream, she is systemically unwell and she has loin tenderness. These findings point to the diagnosis of pyelonephritis.

! Symptoms of a urinary tract infection

- Infant – fever, vomiting, lethargy, irritability, poor feeding
- Older child – frequency, dysuria, abdominal pain or loin pain, fever

---

It is useful to collect two midstream urine specimens before starting intravenous antibiotic therapy, so that the diagnosis of UTI can be confirmed. It is important to avoid contamination by skin flora, by cleaning the external genitalia first and then catching urine cleanly from the middle of the stream (i.e. do not collect the first drops) without the container touching the skin. This should then be sent for microscopy and bacterial culture. Her blood pressure should be measured and, during cannulation, blood should be sent for a full blood count, C-reactive protein, urea, electrolytes, creatinine and blood culture. Further questioning should determine if there have been previous urine infections, recurrent fevers of uncertain origin, a previously diagnosed renal abnormality, a family history of vesicoureteric reflux or constipation. In infants under 6 months and in older children with severe, atypical or recurrent urinary infections, imaging is required to determine if there is an underlying renal abnormality. Leah will therefore require an ultrasound of her urinary tract in the next few days. Prophylactic antibiotics are no longer used routinely after a first urinary tract infection but may be required in children with recurrent urinary infections.

Leah may have an underlying structural renal tract abnormality predisposing to infection. The VACTERL association is the sporadic, non-random, concurrence of at least three of: vertebral, anal, cardiac, tracheo-oesophageal, renal and limb abnormalities. She should also have spinal X-rays to determine the cause of her kyphoscoliosis, e.g. a hemivertebra (see Case 60, p. 183). It would be useful to obtain her previous medical records to find out more about her previous history and investigations.

 KEY POINTS

- Urinalysis should be performed in any unwell, febrile child.
- In infants under 6 months and in older children with severe, atypical or recurrent urinary infections, imaging is required to determine if there is an underlying renal abnormality.

CASE 35: RED URINE

History

Fiona is a 6-year-old girl who presents to the A&E department where her mother states that Fiona's urine has turned red. She has brought a jar of urine which contains what appears to be reddish-brown urine. She has no dysuria, frequency or abdominal pain and there is no history of trauma. She is otherwise well but she and the rest of the family have recently had colds. There have been no nosebleeds or abnormal bruising. She has had no problems with her joints. She had a urinary tract infection at the age of 4 years, but following a normal renal ultrasound she was discharged from clinic. She is on no medication. There is no family history of renal problems but her grandmother has hypertension.

Examination

There is no anaemia. She is apyrexial. There is no skin rash or bruising. There is no oedema of the legs. There are no abdominal signs or joint abnormalities. Blood pressure is 124/80 mmHg. There are no other signs.

INVESTIGATIONS		
		Normal
Haemoglobin	11.7 g/dL	11.5–15.5 g/dL
White cell count	8.7×10^9/L	$4.0–11.0 \times 10^9$/L
Platelets	372×10^9/L	$150–400 \times 10^9$/L
Sodium	137 mmol/L	135–145 mmol/L
Potassium	4.1 mmol/L	3.5–5.0 mmol/L
Urea	11.3 mmol/L	1.8–6.4 mmol/L
Creatinine	145 μmol/L	27–62 μmol/L
Alkaline phosphatase	372 U/L	145–420 U/L
Bilirubin	16 μmol/L	2–26 μmol/L
Alanine aminotransferase (ALT)	32 U/L	10–40 U/L
Albumin	41 g/L	37–50 g/L
Clotting	Normal	
Urine dipstick		
Blood	4+	
Protein	2+	
Leucocytes	1+	
Nitrites	Nil	
Microscopy – red blood cells and red blood cell casts seen		

Questions

- What further investigations should be performed?
- What is the most likely diagnosis?
- What is the treatment?

ANSWER 35

The following investigations should be performed:

- throat swab
- anti-streptolysin O titre (ASOT), C3 and C4 – ASOT is raised and C3 is reduced in post-streptococcal glomerulonephritis
- ESR and ANA – will be abnormal in vasculitides, e.g. SLE
- abdominal X-ray and renal US – will demonstrate normality of kidneys and help exclude calculi.

The most likely diagnosis is a post-streptococcal glomerulonephritis. This condition typically occurs approximately 2 weeks after a streptococcal upper respiratory tract infection (it may also follow a streptococcal skin infection). It can be associated with varying degrees of oliguria and renal failure (in this case there is mild renal failure). The casts indicate renal involvement.

In cases of red urine or blood in the nappy, one should first ensure the blood is from the urinary tract and not from the rectum (e.g. due to constipation) or from the vagina (e.g. periods or abuse). Foods such as beetroot can lead to red urine. Haemoglobinuria due to haemolysis will also lead to red urine which will be dipstick-positive for blood but there will be no red blood cells on microscopy.

The causes of haematuria are:

- urinary tract infection
- nephritis – post-streptococcal glomerulonephritis
  - Henoch–Schönlein purpura
  - IgA nephropathy
  - nephrotic syndrome (20 per cent have haematuria at presentation)
- calculi
- trauma
- haematological – clotting disorders, haemolytic uraemic syndrome
- anatomical causes – polycystic kidneys, hydronephrosis
- tumours, e.g. Wilms' tumour
- drugs, e.g. cyclophosphamide, aspirin
- factitious illness
- recurrent benign haematuria (a diagnosis by elimination).

Treatment is primarily symptomatic. A 10-day course of oral penicillin should be given but this will not alter the natural history of the glomerulonephritis. Fluids should be restricted to 1 L/day and the diet should have no added salt. Frusemide is helpful in cases of hypertension (this girl's blood pressure is greater than the 95th centile for a 6-year-old girl) or oedema and will increase urine output. If hypertension persists, a calcium channel blocker such as amlodipine may be helpful. If heavy proteinuria develops or if renal function deteriorates, a renal opinion should be sought. Indications for dialysis include life-threatening hyperkalaemia and the clinical manifestations of uraemia. Outpatient follow-up will necessitate the monitoring of blood pressure, urea and electrolytes/creatinine and urine dipstick. More than 95 per cent of patients make a complete recovery. Complications include nephrotic range proteinuria and renal failure.

KEY POINTS

- Urinary tract infections, post-streptococcal glomerulonephritis and Henoch–Schönlein purpura account for the majority of cases of haematuria.
- Post-streptococcal glomerulonephritis has a very good prognosis.

CASE 36: A PUFFY FACE

History

Freddie is a 3-year-old boy who presents to the paediatric rapid referral clinic with a 2-day history of puffy eyes. His GP initially prescribed antihistamines but these have not helped. He is otherwise well. He has asthma, which is treated with budesonide 100 μg b.d. and salbutamol two to six puffs 4-hourly as necessary. He is on no other medication. His mother suffers from asthma and hay fever.

Examination

He looks well and is apyrexial. He has puffy eyes and pitting pedal oedema. Pulse is 112 beats/min, blood pressure is 103/70 mmHg and capillary refill is 2 s. There is no abdominal distension, tenderness or organomegaly. However, his scrotum appears oedematous. Respiratory rate is 28 breaths/min and there are no respiratory signs.

INVESTIGATIONS		
		Normal
Haemoglobin	15.2 g/dL	11.5–15.5 g/dL
White cell count	11.7×10^9/L	$4.0–11.0 \times 10^9$/L
Platelets	472×10^9/L	$150–400 \times 10^9$/L
Sodium	142 mmol/L	135–145 mmol/L
Potassium	4.2 mmol/L	3.5–5.0 mmol/L
Urea	6.3 mmol/L	1.8–6.4 mmol/L
Creatinine	59 μmol/L	27–62 μmol/L
Alkaline phosphatase	372 U/L	145–420 U/L
Bilirubin	18 μmol/L	2–26 μmol/L
Alanine aminotransferase (ALT)	37 U/L	10–40 U/L
Albumin	19 g/L	37–50 g/L
Urine dipstick		
Blood, 1+		
Protein, 4+		
Leucocytes, nil		
Nitrites, nil		

Questions

- What is the diagnosis?
- What other investigations should to be performed at presentation?
- What is the treatment?
- What are the complications of this condition?

ANSWER 36

The diagnosis is nephrotic syndrome. This condition consists of the combination of oedema, heavy proteinuria (protein ≥3+ on dipstick), hypoalbuminaemia (albumin <25 g/L, it is only when the albumin falls below this level that one gets oedema) and hyperlipidaemia. In about 20 per cent of cases of nephrotic syndrome there is haematuria. However, urine dipstick are very sensitive and this should be confirmed by sending the urine for microscopy to see if red blood cells or red blood cell casts are visible.

The following investigations should be done:

- Blood
  - cholesterol and triglyceride levels (elevated in nephrotic syndrome)
  - anti-streptolysin O titre (ASOT) and C3/C4 levels to investigate the possibility of post-streptococcal disease
  - antinuclear antibody (ANA), which may be positive in vasculitides such as SLE
  - hepatitis B antibodies if from an at-risk population, as this is a rare cause of nephrotic syndrome
  - measles and *Varicella zoster* antibodies (these are important to know as children who are on immunosuppressive therapy such as steroids are more vulnerable to these conditions)
  - blood culture if febrile
- Urine – microscopy and culture, spot urine protein/creatinine ratio (will be >2 in nephrotic syndrome).

Treatment consists of prednisolone 60 mg/m^2 (maximum daily dose 60 mg) given as a single morning dose for 4 weeks followed by (if in remission, defined as urine dipstick negative or trace for protein on three consecutive days) a prolonged reducing regime. Because of the increased risk of bacterial infections (due to urinary losses of immunoglobulins, immunosuppressive therapy and other factors), most paediatricians administer prophylactic penicillin until the patient is in remission.

Fluid balance is very important. Our patient does not have hypovolaemia, but this should always be assessed, especially if the albumin is very low or if there is vomiting or diarrhoea. Four-hourly observations, including blood pressure, should be done, weight should be assessed once or twice daily, an input/output chart should be kept, and children should be on a low-salt diet.

There are several potential complications. Hypovolaemia may present with non-specific symptoms, such as abdominal pain and vomiting. The haematocrit will be >0.45. It can be treated with 0.9 per cent sodium chloride or 4.5 per cent human albumin 10–20 mL/kg intravenously over 1 hour. Bacterial sepsis is a further important complication. Bacterial peritonitis is the commonest type of infection and *Streptococcus pneumoniae* is the most common organism, but other infections and organisms may also be involved. There is also a risk (2–5 per cent) of thromboembolic events due to hyperviscosity. These may be venous (e.g. renal vein thrombosis) or arterial (e.g. pulmonary embolus).

Approximately 70 per cent of patients relapse (≥2+ proteinuria for three consecutive days or proteinuria with oedema).

 KEY POINTS

- Nephrotic syndrome consists of the combination of oedema, heavy proteinuria, hypoalbuminaemia and hyperlipidaemia.
- Seventy per cent of patients relapse.

CASE 37: A BED WETTER

History

Alvin is a 9-year-old black British boy who has been referred to paediatric outpatients because of bedwetting. He is accompanied by his father. He wets the bed most nights, does not wake up when it happens and there is a large pool of urine. He has no previous medical problems and no recent illnesses. His father says he is unsure if there is any family history of bedwetting. They tried using an enuresis alarm 2 years ago, and the alarm woke him up but he was already wet so they gave up after 1 week. Alvin is quite upset about his bedwetting, particularly because he recently wet the bed when he stayed at a friend's house and has been teased about this at school. Alvin's father is despairing and has started waking him at night to go to toilet, but sometimes he is already wet. He says this is affecting his ability to work and he feels that Alvin is being lazy and should be able to control his bladder at this age.

Examination

His height is 140 cm (75th centile) and his weight is 35 kg (75th centile). His blood pressure is 112/70 mmHg. Cardiovascular, respiratory and abdominal examinations are unremarkable.

🔍 INVESTIGATIONS		
		Normal
Urine analysis		
Leucocytes	Negative	Negative
Nitrites	Negative	Negative
Blood	Negative	Negative
Glucose	Negative	Negative
Specific gravity	1.002	1.002–1.035

Questions
- What further history is required?
- What further examination is necessary?
- What are the options for management?

ANSWER 37

Nocturnal enuresis is defined as involuntary voiding of urine during sleep at least three times per week in a child aged 5 years or older. Approximately 10 per cent of 5-year-olds and 5 per cent of 10-year-olds are affected. It is essential to establish if this is primary or secondary. Primary nocturnal enuresis indicates that he has never achieved dryness at night and three mechanisms may contribute to this: lack of arousal from sleep, bladder instability or low functional bladder capacity, and nocturnal polyuria due to low vasopressin levels. Secondary enuresis indicates that he had previously achieved dryness at night for at least 6 months and something has happened to cause bedwetting again. Secondary causes include constipation, urinary tract infection, diabetes mellitus or psychosocial stresses, such as bullying or a recent parental separation. It is important to establish if there are daytime symptoms of urgency, frequency, dysuria or wetting, which suggest bladder instability or urinary tract infections. An accurate diary of fluid intake and voiding throughout the day is helpful. A family history of bedwetting, renal problems and sickle cell trait/disease (associated with reduced urinary concentrating ability) should be sought.

Examination should include plotting the child's height and weight on a growth chart and a urine analysis. In addition, the genitalia and spine should be inspected for abnormalities, and lower limb neurology should be assessed.

! **Management options for primary nocturnal enuresis**

- Self help measures – regular daytime fluid intake and voiding, avoid caffeinated drinks
- Enuresis clinic support
- Nocturnal polyuria – desmopressin (synthetic analogue of antidiuretic hormone)
- Lack of arousal – enuresis alarm with star chart
- Bladder instability – bladder retraining, anticholinergic medication

---

In this case, there are features of both nocturnal polyuria and lack of arousal from sleep. Unfortunately the father is not sympathetic and unlikely to have the commitment to make an enuresis alarm succeed. In this setting, desmopressin may provide some respite to the family. This will reduce nocturnal urine production. It is important to emphasize early that this is not something Alvin has any control over, that desmopressin is not a solution in the very long term, and that ultimately he may need other methods of treatment. Desmopressin can be withdrawn in a structured fashion, assisted by the use of an enuresis alarm, when the family are ready to support Alvin and invest some effort in his treatment. It may take a long time to achieve consistent dryness through the night. The family may need psychological support.

Desmopressin can cause headache, nausea and abdominal pain, and may be dangerous if there is excessive fluid intake.

⚷ **KEY POINTS**

- Nocturnal enuresis is very common and should only be investigated in children older than 5 years.
- It is essential to establish if nocturnal enuresis is primary or secondary.

CASE 38: HIGH BLOOD PRESSURE

History

Nikita is a 12-year-old Asian girl who is referred to paediatric outpatients by her GP because she has high blood pressure and is overweight. She came to see her GP because she had an ear infection and the GP measured her BP because she is overweight. It was raised and he repeated it a week later when Nikita had recovered and the reading was the same. Nikita is otherwise well but gets headaches about once every 2 weeks. There is no nausea or vomiting. The headaches have been occurring for about 2 years. She had grommets inserted when she was 4 years old. She started her periods 1 year ago and her periods are regular. She is on no medication. Her mother has hypertension.

Examination

Her height is 167 cm (91st centile), weight 85.3 kg (>99.6th centile) and body mass index (BMI) is 30.6 kg/m². Her blood pressure is 146/82 mmHg. There are no dysmorphic features. She has no cardiovascular signs and femoral pulses are palpable. There are pink abdominal striae. There is no organomegaly or abdominal masses. There are no neurological or respiratory signs.

INVESTIGATIONS (Done by the GP)		Normal
Full blood count	Normal	
Sodium	137 mmol/L	135–145 mmol/L
Potassium	4.1 mmol/L	3.5–5.0 mmol/L
Urea	6.2 mmol/L	1.8–6.4 mmol/L
Creatinine	67 μmol/L	44–88 μmol/L
Bone chemistry	Normal	
Liver function tests	Normal	
Thyroid function tests	Normal	
Urine dipstick		
Blood – nil		
Protein – trace		
Leucocytes – nil		
Nitrites – nil		

Questions

- What is the most likely cause of the hypertension in this child?
- What further investigations would you perform?
- What would be your management plan?

ANSWER 38

This child is most likely to have essential (idiopathic) hypertension. This is associated with obesity. Hypertension in pubertal children is most often essential but in prepubertal children there is often a cause.

However, first the diagnosis of hypertension needs to be confirmed. The blood pressure should only be measured after the child has been seated and calm for 5 min. The BP cuff should cover more than three-quarters of the upper right arm and the bladder >50 per cent of the arm circumference (too small a cuff will lead to an artificially high blood pressure). The reading should be repeated at least once. In cases of mild hypertension with no target organ damage (the majority), the blood pressure should be repeated at least three times at weekly intervals to determine if the elevation is sustained. Ideally, 24-hour ambulatory blood pressure monitoring should also be carried out to confirm the diagnosis and to rule out white-coat hypertension. There are charts available with centiles for childrens' blood pressure which are dependent on sex, age and height centile. A systolic or diastolic blood pressure >95th centile denotes hypertension. Headaches can occur in hypertension. In Nikita's case, the cause may be hypertension or the commoner tension type headache. Any obese child can get striae; in Cushing's disease they tend to be purple rather than pink.

! **Causes of hypertension (use the mnemonic – CREED)**

- Cardiological, e.g. coarctation of the aorta
- Renal, e.g. glomerulonephritis, renal artery stenosis
- Essential
- Endocrine, e.g. thyrotoxicosis, Cushing's disease, phaeochromocytoma
- Drugs, e.g. steroids, contraceptive pill, amphetamines

To confirm the diagnosis, 24-hour ambulatory blood pressure monitoring should be performed. Renal disease is the commonest cause of hypertension and a renal ultrasound (ideally with Doppler studies of the renal vessels) should be done. Cardiac pathology is the second commonest cause. The presence of palpable femoral pulses makes a coarctation unlikely. However, an ECG should still be performed to see if the hypertension has led to left ventricular hypertrophy. To investigate the consequences of obesity, a fasting glucose (to rule out type 2 diabetes) and fasting cholesterol and triglyceride levels should be done. Further investigations will depend on confirmation of the hypertension by the ambulatory monitoring and clinical symptomatology.

The management plan should include lifestyle changes. A referral to a dietician should be done and advice given about a low-salt and a low-fat diet. A total of 1 hour of exercise every day should be recommended. If the raised blood pressure is confirmed, a beta-blocker or calcium channel blocker could be used.

  KEY POINTS

- The blood pressure should be measured with the child calm, with the right size of cuff, and be repeated.
- Published centile charts should be consulted.
- Hypertension in pubertal children is most often essential but in prepubertal children there is usually a cause (most commonly renal).

INFECTIONS

CASE 39: FEVER AND A RASH

History

Euan, a 2-year-old boy, is referred to the paediatric day unit by his GP with a history of fever, cough, blocked runny nose and sticky eyes for 6 days. His GP prescribed amoxicillin 2 days ago for otitis media, and that evening he started to develop a rash around his ears and hairline. His parents stopped giving the antibiotics, but the rash continued to spread over most of his body.

The parents report that he has been very miserable and lethargic for the last 5 days. They thought the rash may be an allergic reaction to amoxicillin. He attends nursery but his parents are not aware of any other children there who have been unwell. His parents are well, and he has an older brother who has autism.

Examination

Euan has a temperature of 38.5°C, his heart rate is 115 beats/min, respiratory rate 20/min, and oxygen saturation is 97 per cent in air. He weighs 14 kg (75th centile) and he is miserable and lethargic. He has a widespread maculopapular erythematous rash, which is coalescing over his face, neck and torso. Heart sounds are normal, capillary refill time is 2 s. There is no respiratory distress but he is coughing and there are lots of transmitted upper airway noises heard throughout his chest. His abdomen is normal. His nose is streaming with catarrh and he has a purulent discharge from his right ear. His pharynx is red and he has exudative conjunctivitis.

Questions
- What is the most likely diagnosis?
- What essential piece of history has been omitted?
- What complications may arise from this disease and why has its incidence increased recently in the UK?

ANSWER 39

This is a case of measles. The history is typical, commencing with a catarrhal prodrome phase of fever, conjunctivitis, cough and coryza, preceding development of the rash 3–5 days later. During the catarrhal phase, Koplik's spots may be seen as small white spots on the buccal mucosa. Although pathognomonic of measles, they can be very hard to find and have usually disappeared within 1 day of the rash starting. The rash is maculo-papular and starts around the hairline and behind the ears, spreading downwards across the body. It often becomes confluent on the upper body, resulting in a blotchy appearance. Usually children with measles are very miserable.

! Differential diagnosis of measles	
	Clinical distinguishing features
Kawasaki disease	Not catarrhal
Rubella	Much milder prodrome, occipital lymphadenopathy
Epstein–Barr virus	Tonsillitis, lymphadenopathy, not catarrhal
Roseola infantum (human herpes virus 6, HHV6)	Fever ends as rash appears
Scarlet fever	Pharyngitis or tonsillitis, not catarrhal

An immunization history is an essential part of any paediatric history and no details have been provided here. In fact, Euan had not received the combined measles, mumps and rubella (MMR) vaccine, which is usually given at 13 months of age.

! Complications of measles
• Pneumonia
• Corneal ulceration
• Suppurative otitis media
• Gastroenteritis
• Febrile convulsions
• Encephalomyelitis (rare) and subacute sclerosing panencephalitis (very rare)

Public confidence and uptake of the MMR vaccine fell in the UK following media publicity about a study in 1998 suggesting a link between the vaccine and autism. Despite many publications demonstrating the safety of MMR, and specifically that there is no link to autism, the rate of MMR vaccination in the population fell below that needed to afford herd immunity and cases of measles increased. Measles is a notifiable disease, and prompt notification of suspected cases to the Health Protection Agency allows steps to be taken to minimize further spread and protect those exposed.

KEY POINTS

- Measles has become more common in the UK following a reduction in MMR vaccine uptake.
- Measles has a typical catarrhal phase before onset of the rash.
- The rash evolves in a characteristic fashion, starting around the hairline and behind the ears and spreading downwards.
- Measles is a notifiable disease.

CASE 40: FEVER IN A RETURNING TRAVELLER

History

Michael is a 7-year-old boy brought to the A&E department by his father at 10pm. He has had an intermittent fever and backache for the last 48 hours, has vomited three times, had two loose stools and an episode of violent shivering this evening. He was previously healthy, except for frequent abdominal pain during the last school term, not associated with any change in bowel habit. His parents are originally from Nigeria, although he was born in this country. He has frequently travelled to Nigeria in the summer holidays and returned from his most recent trip 1 week ago. He has received all his routine immunizations according to the UK schedule.

Examination

He looks flushed and withdrawn. His heart rate is 130 beats/min, capillary refill is less than 2 s, respiratory rate 40/min, oxygen saturation 97 per cent in air, and temperature is 39°C. He has no murmurs, breath sounds are normal throughout the chest, he is uncomfortable on abdominal examination, but has no guarding or rebound tenderness. Ears, nose and throat are unremarkable. There is no obvious rash, no lymphadenopathy and no evidence of jaundice.

INVESTIGATIONS		
		Normal
Haemoglobin	11.5 g/dL	11.1–14.7 g/dL
White cell count	17.3 × 10⁹/L	4.5–14.5 × 10⁹/L
Platelets	57 × 10⁹/L	170–450 × 10⁹/L
C-reactive protein	53 mg/L	<5 mg/L
Sodium	133 mmol/L	135–145 mmol/L
Potassium	4.1 mmol/L	3.5–5.6 mmol/L
Urea	2.7 mmol/L	2.5–6.6 mmol/L
Creatinine	42 µmol/L	20–80 µmol/L

Questions
- What other investigations are essential in this child?
- What are the differential diagnoses?
- What further history is important?
- What is the treatment?

ANSWER 40

In any traveller returning from a malaria endemic area, it is absolutely essential to do an urgent thick blood film to look for malaria parasites, and many hospitals now also use a rapid diagnostic test kit to identify the presence of malaria antigens in the blood. It is also important to obtain blood cultures, liver function tests, urine dipstick and, in view of this patient's tachypnoea, a blood gas sample (to look for acidosis) and possibly a chest X-ray. Michael's blood film showed 1 per cent parasitaemia with *Plasmodium falciparum* and the rapid diagnostic test was positive. Malaria cannot be diagnosed or excluded on clinical grounds, and may coexist with other infections. Blood films must be done and three negative films are required to exclude the diagnosis. Thrombocytopenia is commonly seen in malaria, but cannot be relied upon to make the diagnosis.

❗ Non-specific symptoms occuring in children with malaria
• Fever • Diarrhoea • Vomiting • Cough • Tachypnoea • Headache • Lethargy • Coma • Jaundice • Haematuria • Myalgia • Pallor

The differential diagnosis of fever in the returning child traveller can be very wide, including haematuria, malaria, typhoid and all of the causes of childhood fever in their home country (e.g. tonsillitis, myalgia, pneumonia, urinary tract infection, etc). Frequently the cause of the fever is not an unusual or exotic infection at all, even if it was acquired abroad.

An adequate travel history includes details of exactly where the child visited (especially whether urban or rural), what sort of accommodation they stayed in, what activities they did during their visit, and what immunizations and malaria prophylaxis they had. Michael did not take any prophylaxis because his parents felt malaria was not a serious illness.

Treatment should be started promptly, guided by advice from an expert in infectious diseases. A variety of oral treatment options are available for uncomplicated malaria, but intravenous quinine remains the standard treatment for severe disease. Broad-spectrum antibiotic cover should also be given in the case of a seriously unwell child.

KEY POINTS
• Fever in a traveller returning from a malaria-endemic area is malaria until proven otherwise. • Non-specific symptoms should not be interpreted as ruling out the diagnosis. • Prompt initiation of treatment is essential.

CASE 41: STICKY EYES

History

Jenna is a 5-day-old girl who is brought to her GP because she has had sticky eyes for 2 days. The GP notes that there is a purulent discharge filling both eyes, and it is very hard to see the conjunctiva clearly. He refers her to the on-call paediatric team. She was born at term by normal vaginal delivery to a 19-year-old first-time mother after an uneventful pregnancy. Her birth weight was 2.75 kg (ninth centile). Her mother smoked throughout pregnancy and drank some alcohol. She had erratic attendance for antenatal care and had refused antenatal screening blood tests. She was discharged from hospital after 12 hours and the baby has been bottle-fed since.

Examination

Jenna looks healthy apart from swollen eyelids with profuse purulent discharge and erythematous conjunctiva. She weighs 2.8 kg. She is afebrile, with a heart rate of 140/min, a respiratory rate of 35/min, normal heart sounds and normal breath sounds. Her abdomen is soft and the liver is palpable 1 cm below the costal margin. Her anterior fontanelle is normotensive.

INVESTIGATIONS		
		Normal
Haemoglobin	13.3 g/dL	13.4–19.8 g/dL
White cell count	9.1×10^9/L	$6–21 \times 10^9$/L
Platelets	353×10^9/L	$170–500 \times 10^9$/L
C-reactive protein	11 mg/L	<5 mg/L
Microscopy of pus from the eye – pus cells +++; Gram-negative diplococci		

Questions
- What is the diagnosis?
- How should the baby be managed?
- What advice should be given to the mother?

ANSWER 41

Jenna has ophthalmia neonatorum (neonatal conjunctival infection) caused by *Neisseria gonorrhoeae*. The differential diagnosis of sticky eyes in a neonate includes nasolacrimal duct obstruction, *Chlamydia trachomatis*, herpes simplex and other bacterial conjunctivitis (e.g. *Staphylococcus aureus*, *Streptococcus pneumoniae*). Inflammation of the conjunctiva is not seen in nasolacrimal duct obstruction, although the eyes may be sticky. Ophthalmia neonatorum is an emergency and requires prompt management to prevent permanent visual impairment and to treat possible systemic infection.

In cases of ophthalmia neonatorum, it is essential to take adequate microbiological specimens and then commence prompt antibiotic treatment. Swabs for chlamydia are usually different from those used for other bacteria and it is necessary to look for both as chlamydia and gonococcal infections can coexist. Gonococcal ophthalmia neonatorum should be treated with intravenous ceftriaxone or cefotaxime and frequent eye irrigation with saline solution. Many experts would also add antibiotic eye drops. The neonate should be evaluated for disseminated infection, although this is unlikely in this infant, who is afebrile and appears systemically well. Ophthalmia neonatorum is a notifiable disease.

Jenna's mother should be told that this is a sexually transmitted infection (STI), which Jenna has almost certainly acquired from the birth canal. It can cause asymptomatic infection in women, but also causes symptomatic infection of the genital tract, pelvic inflammatory disease and perihepatitis. It is very important that she attends a genitourinary medicine clinic for treatment and screening for other STIs and considers discussing this with her partner(s). It is also important to have a more thorough discussion about her social circumstances and why she declined antenatal screening blood tests.

 KEY POINTS

- Ophthalmia neonatorum requires prompt recognition and systemic treatment.
- Appropriate specimens must be sent for both gonococcus and chlamydia.
- The mother must be advised that she and her partner(s) will require screening.

CASE 42: A PERSISTENT FEVER

History

Ben is a 2-year-old boy who presents to the rapid referral paediatric clinic with a 10 day history of fever, blood shot eyes, a sore throat and a rash. He also has an occasional cough. His mum describes him as being miserable with a poor appetite. There is no history of travel or contact with infections. Ben has already had a 6 day course of amoxyl from his GP that made no difference. He had an inguinal hernia operated on at 2 weeks of age. There is no other medical history of note.

Examination

Temperature 39.8°C. He has bilateral conjunctivitis, erythematous, cracked lips and an erythematous pharynx. There is a non-specific maculopapular rash over the trunk. There is cervical lymphadenopathy with the largest node being 2 cm in diameter, but no lymphadenopathy elsewhere. His chest is clear and there are no other abnormalities.

INVESTIGATIONS		
		Normal
Haemoglobin	10.7 g/dL	10.5–13.5 g/dL
White cell count (WCC)	26.3 × 10^9/L	4.0–11.0 × 10^9/L
Neutrophils	18.2 × 10^9/L	1.7–7.5 × 10^9/L
Platelets	430 × 10^9/L	150–400 × 10^9/L
Sodium	137 mmol/L	135–145 mmol/L
Potassium	3.7 mmol/L	3.5–5.0 mmol/L
Urea	4.2 mmol/L	1.8–6.4 mmol/L
Creatinine	58 μmol/L	27–62 μmol/L
C-reactive protein (CRP)	63 mg/L	<6 mg/L
Erythrocyte sedimentation rate (ESR)	107 mm/hour	0–15 mm/hour

Questions
- What is the likely diagnosis?
- What is the treatment?

ANSWER 42

Fever and rash are very common in paediatrics. Most rashes are non-specific viral rashes but some illnesses are accompanied by typical rashes. For instance, chickenpox is characterized by a maculopapular rash that evolves into vesicles and meningococcal septicaemia by a petechial non-blanching rash.

The most likely diagnosis in this case is Kawasaki's disease which is a vasculitis. This disorder occurs mainly in young children (80 per cent <5 years). It is diagnosed clinically.

Criteria for diagnosis are:

- The presence of a fever for 5 or more days and four of the following five features:
    - non-purulent conjunctivitis
    - cervical lymphadenopathy
    - skin rash
    - erythema of the oral and pharyngeal mucosa
    - erythema and swelling of the hands and feet (followed a week later by skin desquamation).

Accompanying features are a raised WCC, CRP and ESR. In the second week of the illness a thrombocytosis usually develops.

When assessing a child with a prolonged fever (>7 days), the following conditions should be considered.

! **Causes of a prolonged fever**

- Infections, e.g. tuberculosis, HIV
- Malignant diseases, e.g. lymphoma
- Autoimmune diseases, e.g. juvenile idiopathic arthritis
- Miscellaneous, e.g. drugs, inflammatory bowel disease

Treatment consists of an infusion of immunoglobulins on the day of diagnosis, initially high-dose aspirin at anti-inflammatory doses followed by low-dose aspirin at anti-thrombotic doses.

The main complication of this disorder is coronary artery aneurysms that can, in some cases, lead to myocardial infarction and sudden death. A prolonged fever (>16 days), male sex, age <1 year, cardiomegaly, raised inflammatory markers and raised platelets are all risk factors. An echocardiogram at diagnosis and follow-up echocardiograms are required to rule out this complication. The prognosis is related to the cardiac complications. The risk of cardiac complications if treatment with immunoglobulins was commenced within 10 days of diagnosis is <10 per cent.

🔑 **KEY POINTS**

- Kawasaki's disease should be considered in all children with a prolonged fever.
- Treatment consists of immunoglobulins and aspirin.
- The main long-term complication is coronary artery aneurysms.

CASE 43: RECURRENT INFECTIONS

History

Michelle is a 7-year-old girl who presents to the A&E department with a 2-day history of fever, progressively worsening headache, vomiting and neck stiffness. She was born in Zimbabwe and moved to the UK at 2 years of age to live with her aunt, after her mother died from tuberculosis. She was admitted to hospital last year with pneumonia and developed an empyema, which required drainage. *Streptococcus pneumoniae* was isolated from blood cultures at that time. Since then she has had several episodes of otitis media treated by her GP, and has been off school quite frequently. Her aunt is not very sure about which immunizations she has received. There has not been any recent travel.

Examination

Michelle has a temperature of 38.8°C, heart rate 120 beats/min, her blood pressure is 100/65 mmHg, respiratory rate 20/min and her oxygen saturation is 96 per cent in air. Her weight is 17 kg (second centile) and her height is 114 cm (ninth centile). She has multiple enlarged cervical lymph nodes, oral candidiasis, extensive dental caries and suppurative left otitis media. There is no rash, and cardiovascular, respiratory and abdominal examinations are normal. She is alert but uncomfortable, has marked neck rigidity and prefers the lights to be dimmed. There are no other abnormalities found on neurological examination.

! INVESTIGATIONS		
		Normal
Blood		
Haemoglobin	11.3 g/dL	11.1–14.7 g/dL
White cell count	23.8 × 10⁹/L	4.5–14.5 × 10⁹/L
Platelets	400 × 10⁹/L	170–450 × 10⁹/L
C-reactive protein	207 mg/L	<6 mg/L
Glucose	5.5 mmol/L	3.3–5.5 mmol/L
Cerebrospinal fluid		
White cells	1020 × 10⁶/L	<5 × 10⁶/L
Red cells	0	0–2 × 10⁶/L
Protein	2200 mg/L	200–400 mg/L
Glucose	0.9 mmol/L	2.8–4.4 mmol/L
Gram stain	Gram-positive cocci	Negative

Questions

- What is the diagnosis for the acute illness and what is the management?
- What other problems should be considered?
- What other investigations might be appropriate?

ANSWER 43

This child has acute bacterial meningitis, which is most likely to be due to *S. pneumoniae*. This diagnosis is strongly suspected from the acute history and the blood results, and confirmed by the CSF findings (see Case 62, p. **187**). It may have developed secondary to the otitis media. She should be commenced on an appropriate antibiotic (most commonly intravenous ceftriaxone) and on intravenous dexamethasone.

Michelle has a history of recurrent infections with two of these being severe. Any child with unusual, severe, recurrent or persistent infections must be evaluated for the possibility of an underlying immunodeficiency. In this case, recurrent *S. pneumoniae* infections raise concerns about hyposplenism, antibody deficiency and HIV infection. The findings of severe dental caries, oral candidiasis and cervical lymphadenopathy, together with the history of immigration from Zimbabwe and her mother dying from TB, strongly suggest HIV. Testing for HIV is done with informed consent of the person with parental responsibility for the child. If the test is positive, the child will gradually be given information and prepared for disclosure of the diagnosis when they are able to comprehend the implications of having HIV.

!	Examples of factors predisposing to recurrent infections	
	Primary	*Secondary*
	Antibody deficiency	HIV
	Complement deficiency	Immunosuppressive drugs
	Neutropenia	Malnutrition
	Chronic granulomatous disease	Hyposplenism
	Cellular immunodeficiency	Cystic fibrosis
	Ataxia telangiectasia	Anatomical anomalies, e.g. skull base defect

---

 KEY POINTS

- Consider immunodeficiency in all children with unusual, severe, persistent and recurrent infections.
- HIV testing should be part of the assessment of a child with recurrent infections.

CASE 44: UNEXPLAINED WEIGHT LOSS

History

Ehsan is seen in the paediatric clinic with his mother, who speaks little English. He is 12 years old, was born in Afghanistan and moved to the UK as a refugee 3 months ago. He was diagnosed with asthma when he was seen in the A&E department 4 weeks ago, on the basis of a chronic nocturnal cough. Today his mother is more worried about the fact that he has been losing weight and has had a poor appetite since coming to the UK.

Ehsan is using salbutamol and beclometasone inhalers, which have not improved his cough. He has not yet been to school in the UK. He lives with his mother and three younger siblings in a damp two-bedroom flat and his mother has also been coughing a lot over the last month. His father died last year. They are uncertain which immunizations he has received, but he was healthy before coming to the UK. He has been feeling too tired to play games with his siblings for the last 4 weeks and he finds that his clothes are all much looser than when he arrived in the UK. His mother says that he sometimes feels hot, but she has not measured his temperature.

Examination

He is very thin, his height is 153 cm (75th centile) and his weight is 27 kg (second centile). His heart rate is 80 beats/min, his respiratory rate is 26/min, and oxygen saturation is 97 per cent in air. There is no wheeze but there are bronchial breath sounds in the right upper zone of his chest. There is no lymphadenopathy and his cardiovascular and abdominal examinations are unremarkable.

 INVESTIGATIONS

Ehsan's chest radiograph is shown in Figure 44.1.

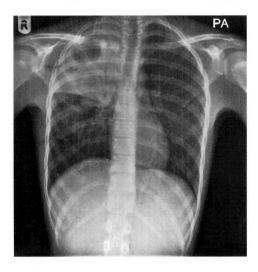

Figure 44.1 Ehsan's chest radiograph.

Questions

- What further history is required?
- What does the chest radiograph show?
- What is the most likely diagnosis?
- What further tests are needed?
- What is the treatment?

ANSWER 44

A history of weight loss with a chronic cough needs to be fully investigated. It is important to ask about the past medical history, family history and contact history with direct
questions about tuberculosis. What happened to this boy's father? (In fact, he died in
Afghanistan after suddenly coughing up a large amount of blood.) Even if the immunization history is unknown, they may know if Ehsan has received the BCG (as this leaves
a distinctive scar) and whether he has ever been treated for TB. Ask about the onset of
the cough, whether it is productive, whether there is bloodstained sputum and if there is
any chest pain or dyspnoea. Ask about exacerbating and relieving factors. Ask when the
weight loss started and whether it is associated with abdominal pain, diarrhoea, malab-
sorptive (bulky, offensive) stools, nausea or vomiting. Also ask about night sweats.

! **Causes of weight losss**

- Inadequate nutrition/neglect
- Gastro-oesophageal reflux
- Coeliac disease
- Inflammatory bowel disease
- Cystic fibrosis
- Anorexia nervosa
- Cardiac failure
- Chronic renal failure
- Diabetes mellitus
- Malignancy
- Infections, e.g. tuberculosis, HIV

The chest radiograph shows dense consolidation and cavitation in the right upper lobe.
The most likely diagnosis is pulmonary tuberculosis. Ehsan's father probably died from
pulmonary tuberculosis and Ehsan's mother probably also has pulmonary tuberculosis.

Ehsan will require admission for investigation and treatment, with isolation whilst he
may have mycobacteria in his sputum. The possibility of multidrug-resistant TB should
be considered in view of his recent immigration from Afghanistan.

The gold standard for diagnosis of tuberculosis is culture of the mycobacteria from clinical specimens. Unfortunately this is much more difficult to achieve in children than in
adults, and only possible in less than 50 per cent of cases. More often the diagnosis is
based on suggestive clinical and radiological features, history of exposure to TB, and
results of tuberculin skin testing (TST). Interpretation of the TST is affected by prior
BCG vaccination, and new tests based on the release of interferon-gamma from blood
mononuclear cells in response to antigens present in TB but not in BCG may aid diagnosis further. Ehsan will require a tuberculin skin test, sputum to be collected for microscopy and culture, erythrocyte sedimentation rate, C-reactive protein, full blood count
and liver function tests. It is more likely that his sputum will show acid-fast bacilli on
microscopy, because he has cavitating pulmonary disease. Cavities are often teeming
with mycobacteria. This presentation would be much rarer in younger children, who
rarely have cavitating disease. If he is unable to expectorate sputum by himself, techniques to induce sputum production may be attempted, and gastric aspirates may be sent
for mycobacterial culture (but their positive yield is much lower). Drug sensitivity testing

will be needed on cultured specimens. Ehsan and his mother should be counselled for an HIV test, because HIV is an important risk factor for development of TB.

Standard treatment for pulmonary tuberculosis should commence with four drugs: isoniazid, rifampicin, ethambutol and pyrazinamide. Pyridoxine is often given to adolescents to reduce the risk of isoniazid causing peripheral neuropathy. The rest of the family will need to be screened for evidence of active or latent tuberculosis. Latent tuberculosis occurs when a person has been infected with TB, but, rather than causing disease, the mycobacteria become dormant. Individuals with latent tuberculosis are generally not infectious to others but are at risk of developing active tuberculosis in the future. Chemoprophylaxis (a course of one or two anti-tuberculous drugs) is advised for latent infection.

Tuberculosis is a notifiable disease and the incidence has been increasing in the UK. The majority of cases occur in non-UK-born young adults.

 KEY POINTS

- Suspicion of tuberculosis should be high in children from high-incidence countries with a compatible clinical history.
- The likelihood of obtaining a positive sputum smear or culture in children with pulmonary tuberculosis is much lower than in adults.
- Diagnosis of tuberculosis is often made on the basis of likelihood of exposure, clinical and radiological findings and tuberculin skin testing.

DERMATOLOGY

CASE 45: AN ITCHY RASH

History
Diamond is a 3-year-old boy who presents to his GP with an itchy rash that he has had for 4 days. He is otherwise well. He had bronchiolitis at the age of 4 months but has had no other diseases. He is not on any medication. His 5-year-old brother has eczema and his father has hay fever. He attends nursery three times a week. The family live in a one-bedroom flat which is damp. His father smokes 20 cigarettes a day.

Examination
He is systemically well and apyrexial. He is very itchy, cannot stop scratching and has obvious linear scratch marks. He has papules, pustules with some associated crusting and a few vesicles. The fingers, hands, flexor surfaces of the arms, axilla and feet seem to be the worst affected areas but there are also lesions around the umbilicus and on the face.

Questions
- What is the most likely diagnosis?
- What is the differential diagnosis of an itchy rash in a child?
- What is the treatment?

ANSWER 45

The most likely diagnosis is scabies. This is caused by the mite *Sarcoptes scabiei* and is highly contagious. Intense itching is typical. However, in children under 1 year this may present as irritability. A history of contact may be present. The classic features are burrows, papules, vesicles and pustules. Thread-like, linear burrows, typically in the finger webs and wrists, are pathognomonic but are often difficult to see. Definitive diagnosis involves removal of the mite from the burrow and examination under the microscope, but this, too, is difficult. Secondary bacterial infection due to scratching is common. In infants, the rash usually affects the palms, soles, axilla and scalp. In older children, lesions typically involve the web space between the fingers, the flexor aspects of the wrist and arm, the axilla and the waistline. The face is rarely involved in those over 5 years of age. Other areas of the body can also be affected. Although there is a strong family history of atopy, the patient has never had eczema and it would be unusual for eczema to present for the first time at this age in this way.

Common causes of an itchy rash in a child are:

- eczema – very common, often involves face, elbow and knee flexures
- seborrhoeic dermatitis – affects infants, often in association with cradle cap
- scabies – itchy where mite has burrowed
- insect bites – affects uncovered areas such as arms and legs
- drug allergy
- urticaria – idiopathic or secondary to allergens, consists of wheal (raised and white) and flare (red)
- fungal infections – e.g. tinea capitis or tinea pedis (athlete's foot)
- chickenpox.

Treatment consists of the application of scabicidal medication, e.g. permethrin. Family members and 'kissing contacts' should also be treated. Topical or oral antibiotics may also be required to treat secondary bacterial infection. Oral antihistamines and topical steroids, e.g. 1 per cent hydrocortisone, may be needed to help treat the itching. All clothing and bed linen should be laundered to remove eggs and mites. It can take 4–6 weeks for the itching to resolve. If lesions are still present at this time, persistent infection or reinfection should be suspected and treatment may need repeating.

 KEY POINTS

- Scabies infestation causes severe itching.
- The classic features are linear burrows, papules, vesicles and pustules.
- The treatment of choice is permethrin.

CASE 46: DETERIORATING ECZEMA

History

George is a 2-year-old boy who presents to the paediatric rapid referral clinic with a worsening of his eczema. The latter was diagnosed by the GP when he was 6 months old. He has been treated with a variety of emollients and topical steroids which are applied on an intermittent, as-required basis. The parents report that over the last 3 days the eczema has gradually deteriorated and also become more itchy. George also has asthma which is treated with inhaled budesonide twice a day and inhaled salbutamol on an as-required basis. His mother had eczema as a child but grew out of it and his father has hay fever.

Examination

George is well hydrated. His temperature is 38.3°C, he is itchy and miserable. He has widespread eczema all over his body, which is worst on his face, hands and arms where the skin feels moist (see Fig. 46.1). A number of vesicles and some punched-out lesions can be seen on the face, hands and arms. There are also pustules and some areas of honey-coloured crusting in those areas. In some areas the lesions have coalesced. The marked scratching that has taken place makes the exact nature of the lesions more difficult to determine. His eyes are puffy and there are some surrounding lesions. The eyes themselves appear normal but are difficult to assess fully. There is cervical, axillary and inguinal lymphadenopathy. His chest is clear.

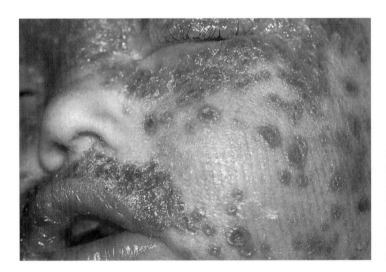

Figure 46.1 Eczema on George's face. (Reproduced with kind permission from Kane KSM *et al.*, *Color Atlas and Synopsis of Pediatric Dermatology*, McGraw Hill, 2002.)

🔍 **INVESTIGATIONS**		
		Normal
Haemoglobin	10.2 g/dL	10.5–14.0 g/dL
White cell count (WCC)	23.2×10^9/L	$5.0–15.0 \times 10^9$/L
Neutrophils	9.2×10^9/L	$1.5–8.0 \times 10^9$/L
Lymphocytes	14.0×10^9/L	$4.0–10.0 \times 10^9$/L
Platelets	392×10^9/L	$150–400 \times 10^9$/L
Urea and electrolytes	Normal	
C-reactive protein (CRP)	116 mg/L	<6 mg/L

Questions

- What further investigations are important?
- What is the diagnosis?
- What is the treatment?

ANSWER 46

A blood culture should have been done at the same time as the other blood tests, as there is a small possibility that he may have a septicaemia. Skin swabs should be taken for bacteriology and virology (virology swabs require special viral medium).

The diagnosis is eczema herpeticum with superadded bacterial infection. It would be worth asking if the child has had similar previous episodes or if anyone in the family has herpetic cold sores. Eczema herpeticum is caused by herpes simplex virus infection of eczematous skin. The infection spreads along the skin and haematogenously. Vesicles and pustules occur and these may coalesce, erode the skin and become haemorrhagic and crusted. The lesions can disseminate rapidly and may cause life-threatening infection. Eczema herpeticum may also affect the conjunctiva and cornea and can cause a keratitis that, if left untreated, may lead to blindness. The diagnosis is sometimes made when a patient fails to respond to antibacterial therapy. The raised temperature, WCC and CRP indicate that the infection is severe, and the lymphocytosis is suggestive of a viral infection. The diagnosis can be made by microscopy, culture or viral PCR.

Bacterial infection can also lead to an acute deterioration in eczema (and is more common than herpetic infection). The pathogen is usually *Staphylococcus aureus* and occasionally *Streptococcus*. Staphylococcal infection can lead to honey-coloured crusting, as in this case. In our case, the secondary bacterial infection is most likely to be due to scratching, leading to the *Staphylococcus* that often colonizes the skin, causing infection.

In some cases it can be difficult to determine if the eczema has been infected by bacteria or viruses and both need to be treated.

The lymphadenopathy is secondary to the infected eczema.

In some cases of widespread infected eczema, there can be marked fluid loss from the skin, which may be exacerbated in the presence of a temperature. In this case the patient is well hydrated, but hydration should be carefully monitored (the situation is somewhat analogous to fluid loss in a burn). Intravenous acyclovir should be administered. If there is any concern about possible eye involvement, as in this case, an urgent ophthalmic opinion should be sought. In addition, intravenous antibiotics (e.g. co-amoxiclav) should be given because of the superadded bacterial skin infection and possible septicaemia. Analgesics, antipyretics and anti-pruritic agents, i.e. antihistamines, should be prescribed. Topical treatment with steroids and other immunosuppressants (e.g. tacrolimus) should be discontinued (this is in contrast to bacterial infections alone when steroid creams are usually continued alongside the antibiotic). Topical treatments can usually be restarted after 1 week when the patient has improved.

 KEY POINTS

- Herpetic infection can lead to severe worsening of eczema (eczema herpeticum).
- Bacterial infection is the commonest cause for an acute deterioration in eczema, with the commonest pathogen being *Staphylococcus aureus*.

CASE 47: AN INFANT WITH BLISTERS

History

Amy is an 8-day-old infant referred to the paediatric day unit by the midwife. In the past 24 hours she has developed several blisters in the nappy area plus a few on her trunk and arms. Amy was born at 38 weeks' gestation, following an uneventful pregnancy, to healthy, unrelated parents. There were no risk factors for infection (e.g. prolonged rupture of membranes). She is their first baby. Her mother has quite severe eczema and asthma. Amy is breast-feeding well and has regained her birth weight.

Examination

Amy looks generally well. Her temperature is 36.8°C. There are no dysmorphic features. Her pulse is 130 beats/min and her capillary refill time <2 s. Scattered over her skin (see Fig. 47.1) in the described distribution she has several flaccid, transparent, cloudy, fluid-filled bullae of varying size from 2 to 15 mm in diameter. One or two have ruptured, leaving a shallow, moist erosion.

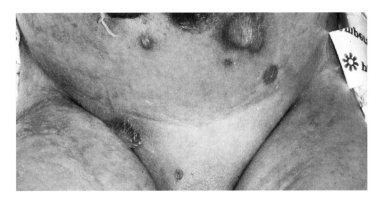

Figure 47.1 Amy's skin.

Amy also has a 5-mm-diameter soft glistening pink lesion within the umbilicus where the cord has dropped off. It bleeds a little on contact and there is a small blood stain on her nappy. Examination of the cardiovascular, respiratory and abdominal systems is unremarkable. Her anterior fontanelle is soft. She handles well and has normal tone and primitive reflexes.

$\mathcal{P}$ INVESTIGATIONS		
		Normal
Haemoglobin	14.6 g/dL	13–21 g/dL
WCC	13.3 × 10⁹/L	6–22 × 10⁹/L
Platelets	235 × 10⁹/L	150–400 × 10⁹/L
Sodium	138 mmol/L	134–146 mmol/L
Potassium	4.4 mmol/L	3.0–7.0 mmol/L
Urea	2.2 mmol/L	1.8–6.4 mmol/L
Creatinine	46 μmol/L	27–62 μmol/L
CRP	<6 mg/L	<6 mg/L

Questions
- What is the most likely cause of the bullae?
- What is the management?
- What is the umbilical lesion likely to be, and how would you treat it?

ANSWER

These flaccid, fragile blisters are characteristic of bullous impetigo. This is the localized presentation of the staphylococcal scalded-skin syndrome and patients are otherwise well. At the other end of the spectrum are those who present with generalized cutaneous involvement and systemic illness. Both are caused by *Staphylococcus aureus,* most of which are from phage group 2. In bullous impetigo the organism can be cultured from the lesions but the systemic form is mediated by exfoliative toxins and swabs are sterile.

The common weepy, golden, crusty forms of impetigo start on skin that has been damaged, e.g. by insect bites, chickenpox or abrasions. It spreads easily to other sites and to other children. The causative organism is also usually *Staphylococcus aureus* but generally not from phage group 2. Group A β-haemolytic *Streptococcus* can also cause impetigo. Patients with eczema are at increased risk of infective exacerbations due to these organisms. It is likely that this baby's infection was transmitted from her mother, either because of her eczema or because she has mastitis.

A much rarer cause of blistering in the neonatal period is epidermolysis bullosa. There are several different types that differ in severity, clinical features, distribution and inheritance patterns, but all are characterized by blisters that develop with trauma and are exacerbated in warm weather. Blisters present at birth would be strongly supportive of this diagnosis.

Treatment is with a β-lactamase-resistant antibiotic such as co-amoxiclav. This infant is well and so the oral route can be safely used whilst monitoring for a satisfactory response. In systemic scalded skin syndrome, antibiotics are administered parenterally. Such patients need careful monitoring because they are at risk of significant heat and fluid losses. They also require adequate pain relief.

The umbilical lesion is likely to be a granuloma. The umbilical cord usually dries and separates within 6–8 days after birth and the surface epithelializes. Where this is incomplete or there is mild infection, granulation tissue can develop and persist. A granuloma is not painful. A number of treatments are available, including cauterization using a silver nitrate stick. This can be repeated once a week until the lesion has resolved. It is crucial to differentiate the common umbilical granuloma from the rare umbilical polyp which results from persistence of the omphalomesenteric duct or the urachus. If it communicates with the ileum or bladder, there may a faeculant or urinary discharge. Treatment is surgical.

 KEY POINTS

- Skin infections due to *Staphyococcus aureus* have a range of presentations from mild, localized lesions to severe, systemic infections.
- Blistering present at birth is likely to be due to epidermolysis bullosa.

HAEMATOLOGY

CASE 48: A PALE CHILD

History

Sarah is a 4-year-old girl who is referred to the paediatric day unit by her GP with a 2-day history of widespread bruising. She has also had two nosebleeds in the preceding 24 hours. There are no known injuries, although her mother says she is quite 'hectic', especially when playing with her younger brother. They both had a cold and a sore throat 2 weeks previously. She is otherwise very well. There is no significant past medical or family history and she is on no medication.

Examination

Sarah is drawing pictures and is cheerful and cooperative. She has no dysmorphic features. Her height and weight are on the 25th centiles. There is no jaundice and she is afebrile. She is pale and clinically anaemic with a few <1.0 cm lymph nodes in the cervical and inguinal regions. There is widespread bruising mainly on her limbs but no evidence of active bleeding. There is no hepatosplenomegaly. Her pulse is 96 beats/min and both heart sounds are normal. She has a grade 2/6 ejection systolic murmur. Examination of the respiratory system is normal.

🔍 INVESTIGATIONS		
		Normal
Haemoglobin	6.2 g/dL	11.5–15.5 g/dL
White cell count	1.2 × 10⁹/L	6.0–17.5 × 10⁹/L
Neutrophils	0.2 × 10⁹/L	3.0–5.8 × 10⁹/L
Lymphocytes	0.8 × 10⁹/L	1.5–3.0 × 10⁹/L
Platelets	6 × 10⁹/L	150–400 × 10⁹/L
Blood film	No blasts	
Prothrombin time	12 s	11–15 s
Partial thromboplastin time	32 s	25–35 s
Urea and electrolytes	Normal	
Liver function tests	Normal	
C-reactive protein	<6 mg/L	<6 mg/L

Questions
- What is the differential diagnosis?
- What investigations are indicated?
- What are her major current risks?

ANSWER 48

Sarah has pancytopenia, loss of all bone marrow (BM) elements. This is not a diagnosis and needs further investigation.

! **Differential diagnosis of pancytopenia**

Bone marrow failure
- **Inherited** – all rare. Commonest is Fanconi's anaemia. Excess chromosome breaks. Defective DNA repair, decreased cell survival and susceptible to oxidant stress. Associated physical abnormalities, e.g. skeletal (absent thumbs), short stature. Only cure is a BM transplant.
- **Acquired**
  - viral, e.g. hepatitis, herpes, Epstein–Barr
  - drugs – idiosyncratic, e.g. chloramphenicol, anticonvulsants, or predictable, e.g. chemotherapy; >80 per cent are 'idiopathic aplastic anaemia'.

Bone marrow infiltration
- Malignancy, e.g. leukaemia or neuroblastoma. Rarely myelofibrosis and myelodysplasia.

Bone marrow infiltration causes marrow expansion and pain unless it is slowly progressive as in myelofibrosis. There are also likely to be other symptoms and signs, e.g. lymphaden-opathy or hepatosplenomegaly in leukaemia. Significantly enlarged lymph nodes are usually >1 cm in diameter. Despite her pallor, this child is playing happily, making BM failure more likely. About 20 per cent of patients with inherited pancytopenias have none of the associated features so an inherited cause cannot be excluded clinically, but these conditions are rare. This girl probably has an acquired pancytopenia – probably idiopathic aplastic anaemia (AA). Most cases appear to be caused by activated T-lymphocytes, producing cytokines that suppress haematopoiesis. Her mild tachycardia and murmur are most likely due to a hyperdynamic circulation secondary to anaemia. An echocardiogram may be indicated if it does not disappear or diminish following transfusion.

! **Investigation of pancytopenia**

- Blood film – detailed morphology of all cell lines
- Red cell indices – the anaemia in AA is normocytic or mildly macrocytic
- Reticulocytes – <20 × 10^9/L suggests severe aplastic anaemia
- Viral titres – hepatitis, Epstein–Barr, parvovirus (usually causes red cell aplasia)
- Chromosomes for breakage analysis
- BM aspirate and trephine – to assess morphology and cellularity of the cells and to exclude infiltration. In AA it is hypocellular but the remaining cells are normal

---

Management pending a diagnosis and treatment is supportive. Haemorrhage and infection are her two major risks. However, there is a danger with multiple platelet transfusions of developing antibodies (alloimmunization). These can cause a typical transfusion reaction with fevers and rigors, but more importantly can diminish the increment in platelet count. This risk is minimized by restricting transfusions to episodes of active bleeding and/or a platelet count of <5 × 10^9/L. Neutropenia, especially if prolonged, puts her at risk of serious life-threatening bacterial infections and the family should be given instructions about regular monitoring of her temperature and when to seek advice.

Spontaneous recovery of idiopathic aplastic anaemia is rare. The decision to embark on definitive treatment depends upon the severity. BM transplant (BMT) offers the best chance for those with a matched sibling donor. Otherwise, immunosuppressive treatment with antithymocyte globulin and cyclosporin is the main alternative. If this fails, a matched, unrelated-donor BMT is the only option.

KEY POINTS

- Pancytopenia can be due to bone marrow failure or bone marrow infiltration.
- The most important risks from pancytopenia are bleeding and infection.

CASE 49: EASY BRUISING

History

Ahmed is a 2-year-old boy who presents to the paediatric rapid referral clinic with easy bruising. His mother states that over the last 2 days bruises have been appearing on his body spontaneously or with minimal trauma and that he also had two short nose bleeds the previous day. He is otherwise well but his mother says that he had a cold about 2 weeks ago. He has had no previous illnesses but had a circumcision at 2 months of age for religious reasons with no excessive bleeding. He is on no medication. There is no family history of bleeding disorders.

Examination

He is well, playing and apyrexial. There is no pallor. He has widespread purpura and bruising over the flexor and extensor surfaces of all four limbs, trunk and face. There is some blood crusted around his nose. There is no lymphadenopathy or hepatosplenomegaly. There are no respiratory or cardiological signs and there are no joint abnormalities.

INVESTIGATIONS		
		Normal
Haemoglobin	10.2 g/dL	10.5–14.0 g/dL
White cell count	9.6×10^9/L	$5.0–15.0 \times 10^9$/L
Neutrophils	4.2×10^9/L	$1.7–7.5 \times 10^9$/L
Platelets	6×10^9/L	$150–400 \times 10^9$/L
Clotting screen	Normal	
Urea and electrolytes	Normal	
C-reactive protein	5 mg/L	<6 mg/L

Blood film – large (young) platelets; no blasts seen
Urine dipstick
  Blood – negative
  Protein – negative
  Leucocytes – negative
  Nitrites – negative

Questions

- What is the diagnosis?
- What are the causes of purpura in a child?
- Are any further investigations necessary?
- What is the treatment?

ANSWER 49

The diagnosis is idiopathic thrombocytopenia purpura (ITP). This condition is caused by antibodies to platelets. The history of a viral infection 2 weeks prior to the onset of the ITP is typical, as is the isolated, very low platelet count in an otherwise well child.

! **Causes of purpura in a child**
• Infections • Thrombocytopenia secondary to ITP, leukaemia or chemotherapy • Henoch–Schönlein purpura (HSP) and other vasculitides • Vomiting or coughing • Trauma • Clotting disorders • Drugs, e.g. steroids

Meningococcal septicaemia is an important cause of purpura. However, the absence of a temperature and the normal inflammatory markers make this diagnosis unlikely. Viral infections, e.g. cytomegalovirus, can cause purpura. The lesions are usually small ($\leq 2\,mm$) and the diagnosis is often made by elimination. The absence of signs such as hepatosplenomegaly and blasts in the film makes leukaemia unlikely. HSP is characterized by a purpuric rash on the extensor surfaces of the lower limbs, joint swelling and blood and/or protein in the urine. Children with vomiting and/or coughing can get purpura in the drainage distribution of the superior vena cava. Accidental or non-accidental trauma does not present with generalized purpura. Clotting disorders more frequently present with haemarthrosis.

No further investigations are required. A bone marrow examination is only indicated if there are atypical clinical features which suggest possible leukaemia. It should also be performed prior to steroid treatment to definitely exclude leukaemia that may be partially treated by steroids.

Treatment is controversial. Most doctors would not treat Ahmed. Approximately 4 per cent of children with ITP have serious symptoms such as severe epistaxis or gastrointestinal bleeding. The most serious complication is an intracranial haemorrhage, the incidence of which is 0.1–0.5 per cent.

The indications for treatment are based on symptoms and not on the platelet count alone. If the child has mucous membrane bleeding and extensive cutaneous symptoms, prednisolone should be administered. Intravenous immunoglobulin can raise the platelet count more rapidly than steroids. However, it carries the risks of pooled blood products and has side-effects, e.g. headache. It should be reserved for the emergency treatment of patients with serious bleeding.

Platelet transfusions are only indicated in the case of an intracranial haemorrhage or to treat life-threatening bleeding. Splenectomy is rarely needed.

Activities with a high risk of trauma should be avoided. Medication, such as ibuprofen, that can affect platelet function should also be avoided.

A repeat full blood count should be performed at 7–10 days to ensure that there is no evolving bone marrow disorder, e.g. aplasia. ITP is usually a self-limiting disorder. Fifty per cent resolve in 2 months, 75 per cent in 4 months and 90 per cent in 6 months.

KEY POINTS

- Treatment in ITP should be guided by symptoms rather than the platelet count.
- The most serious complication is an intracranial haemorrhage.
- Meningococcal septicaemia is an important cause of purpura that requires urgent treatment.

CASE 50: A CHILD WITH CHEST PAIN

History
Rebekah is a 14-year-old Afro-Caribbean girl who presents to the A&E department complaining of pain in her chest and back. Her pain started this morning and has been worsening throughout the day, despite taking paracetamol, ibuprofen and codeine phosphate. She is finding it difficult to breath deeply and the pain is worse on inspiration. She has HbSS sickle cell disease and has been admitted to hospital three times in the last month with painful crises.

Examination
Rebekah's temperature is 38.8°C, her heart rate is 120 beats/min, blood pressure 135/85 mmHg, respiratory rate 40 breaths/min, and oxygen saturation 91 per cent in air. She is in pain and unable to take a deep breath. There are bronchial breath sounds at both lung bases. Heart sounds are normal. Her abdomen is soft and non-tender and her ears and throat are unremarkable.

INVESTIGATIONS		
		Normal
Haemoglobin	7.7 g/dL	12.1–15.1 g/dL
White cell count	19.9×10^9/L	$4.5–13 \times 10^9$/L
Platelets	227×10^9/L	$180–430 \times 10^9$/L
Neutrophils	12.8×10^9/L	$1.5–6.0 \times 10^9$/L
Urea and electrolytes/creatinine	Normal	
Bilirubin	56 mmol/L	1.7–26 mmol/L
Alkaline phosphatase	118 IU/dL	25–125 IU/dL
Aspartate aminotransferase	40 IU/dL	10–45 IU/dL
C-reactive protein	127 mg/L	<5 mg/L
Chest radiograph – see Figure 50.1		

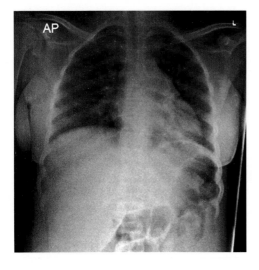

Figure 50.1 Rebekah's initial chest radiograph.

Questions

- What is the most likely cause of the Rebekah's chest pain?
- How should this be managed?
- What other complications can occur in children with sickle cell disease?
- How can infections be prevented in children with sickle cell disease?

ANSWER 50

Rebekah has acute sickle chest syndrome. Thrombosis, infection and fat embolism to the lung produce a syndrome of pleuritic chest pain, shortness of breath and fever. The pathology often evolves from the lung bases and produces consolidation, which may be clinically apparent before radiographic changes appear. Hypoxia is a frequent feature, and failure to recognize and manage this syndrome aggressively may lead to a rapid deterioration. Compare the initial chest radiograph (which shows just a small patch of consolidation in the left lower lobe behind the heart) with the one taken 2 days later (which shows more extensive bi-basal consolidation – see Fig. 50.2).

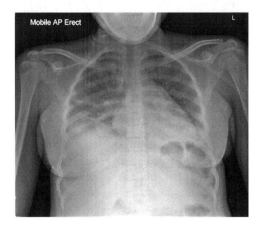

Figure 50.2 Rebekah's chest radiograph 2 days later.

Sickling of red blood cells and their sequestration in vessels is exacerbated by dehydration, hypoxia and acidosis, so these factors need to be corrected with hyperhydration and supplemental oxygen. Adequate analgesia (often intravenous morphine) and physiotherapy help the patient to breathe deeply enough to ventilate the affected areas of the lungs. Empirical antibiotic treatment should be started, e.g. co-amoxiclav and clarithromycin. Children with acute sickle chest syndrome should be discussed with a senior paediatrician and a haematologist. If they deteriorate, they may require ventilatory support (continuous positive airways pressure (CPAP) or intubation and ventilation). A top-up or exchange blood transfusion may also be needed to reduce the percentage of sickling red blood cells.

!	Complications of sickle cell disease in children
	• Painful crises, avascular necrosis of the hips and shoulders • Chest syndrome, abdominal syndrome, girdle syndrome • Splenic sequestration, aplastic anaemic crisis • Stroke, retinal vein occlusion • Priapism, haematuria, enuresis, chronic renal failure • Pigment gallstones, cholecystitis, biliary colic • Hyposplenism, sepsis, osteomyelitis • Delayed puberty

Children with sickle cell disease develop hyposplenism, which makes them particularly vulnerable to infection with encapsulated bacteria such as *Haemophilus influenzae* and *Streptococcus pneumoniae*. They should receive all routine immunizations, pneumococcal polysaccharide vaccine, and regular penicillin V prophylaxis. Hepatitis B vaccine is recommended, and if they travel to a malaria-endemic area, it is essential they take adequate prophylaxis.

 KEY POINTS

- Sickle chest syndrome is an emergency. Early recognition and treatment can prevent severe consequences.
- Children with sickle cell disease are vulnerable to infections with encapsulated bacteria.
- Complications of sickle cell disease can affect any organ.

ONCOLOGY

History

Christopher is a 3-year-old boy who presents to the children's day unit via his GP. The previous evening his mother noticed a lump in his abdomen while drying him after a bath. He has no urinary symptoms and his bowels open normally twice daily. He is otherwise entirely fit and well, and there is no other history of note.

Examination

Christopher is generally healthy with no anaemia, jaundice or lymphadenopathy. His height and weight are on the 75th centile. His blood pressure is 115/75 mmHg. Both heart sounds are normal with no murmurs and his chest is clear. In his abdomen there is a 12-cm-diameter smooth, firm mass in the right flank that extends across the midline. There is no hepatosplenomegaly. The external genitalia are normal.

INVESTIGATIONS		
		Normal
Haemoglobin	11.7 g/dL	11.5–15.5 g/dL
White cell count	8.4×10^9/L	$5.5–15.5 \times 10^9$/L
Platelets	365×10^9/L	$150–400 \times 10^9$/L
Sodium	139 mmol/L	138–146 mmol/L
Potassium	4.3 mmol/L	3.5–5.0 mmol/L
Urea	2.0 mmol/L	1.8–6.4 mmol/L
Creatinine	45 μmol/L	27–62 μmol/L
C-reactive protein	<6 mg/L	<6 mg/L
Midstream urine	>10 red cells	
	1–10 white cells	
	No growth	

Abdominal ultrasound – there is an 11 cm, apparently well-capsulated, solid heterogeneous mass arising from the right kidney. There is no evidence of calcification

Questions

- What is the commonest cause of an abdominal mass in childhood?
- What is the most likely diagnosis in this case?
- Where should he be managed?
- What complication has arisen?

ANSWER 51

The commonest cause of an abdominal mass – occasionally huge – in childhood is faeces. It is characteristically craggy, mobile and in the lower abdomen. However, abdominal masses in children should be assumed to be malignant until proven otherwise, and if there is any doubt, imaging with ultrasound is required.

In an otherwise healthy asymptomatic child, the most likely diagnosis is a Wilms' tumour or nephroblastoma, a neoplasm of the kidney comprising approximately 6 per cent of childhood cancers; 7 per cent are bilateral. It is not unusual for these to present after parents have found the mass incidentally. Wilms' tumours may be associated with hemihypertrophy, aniridia (hypoplastic iris commonly associated with macular and optic nerve hypoplasia) and other congenital abnormalities, usually of the genitourinary tract. Children with Beckwith–Wiedemann syndrome (mutations at 11p15.5, hemihypertrophy, macroglossia and visceromegaly) have such an increased risk of Wilms' (approximately 4 per cent) that they are screened regularly during early childhood.

The main differential diagnosis is neuroblastoma (NB) – an embryonal cancer of the peripheral sympathetic nervous system. Most arise in the abdomen either in an adrenal gland or in the retroperitoneal sympathetic ganglia. The mass usually causes discomfort. Sadly, children with NB often present with symptoms of metastatic spread, such as fever, bone pain, irritability and weight loss – unusual in Wilms'. Tumour markers and imaging help distinguish the two. Ninety-five per cent of NB patients have raised urine vanillylmandelic acid (VMA) and homovanillic acid (HVA). Unlike NB, Wilms' tumours rarely calcify.

Surgery is the mainstay of treatment for Wilms' tumour with pre- and post-surgery chemotherapy and radiotherapy depending on the stage. The prognosis for Wilms' is excellent, with stage 1–3 patients having an overall cure rate of 88–98 per cent. Those with stage 4 disease, with distant metastases, have a poorer but still relatively favourable prognosis of about 75 per cent.

There is good evidence that prognosis in all childhood cancers improves in children managed by specialist units, although some care can be local on a 'shared care' basis. Centralization of care, multidisciplinary teams, entry into randomized controlled trials and the use of national or international protocols have steadily improved the prognosis in all childhood cancers.

His BP is high for a child of his age. Children dislike having their BP measured so it can be difficult to measure accurately. There are electronic devices commonly in use but their results should be interpreted with caution and every effort made to measure BP with standard equipment. The cuff width should be at least two-thirds of the distance from the elbow to the shoulder. Normative ranges according to sex, age and height centile exist for children and adolescents. They are presented as percentiles, with the 95th percentile defining hypertension. In Wilms' tumour, BP is often raised at presentation, probably due to ischaemia. It may persist for several months even after the primary has been removed and may need drug treatment.

KEY POINTS

- Abdominal masses in children are malignant until proven otherwise.
- Wilms' tumour can be associated with congenital anomalies.
- The care of all children with cancer should be coordinated by specialist centres.

CASE 52: AN UNSTEADY CHILD

History

Toby is a 4.5-year-old boy referred to children's outpatients by his GP with a history of apparent stiffness in his neck. About 6 weeks previously he complained of a 'dizzy head' and became reluctant to walk home after school. Subsequently he seemed to find it difficult to look upwards but seemed fine when looking from side to side. He has also been rubbing his head and crying. In the past 3 weeks Toby has had several episodes of vomiting and at the time holds his neck in pain. There have been no other gastrointestinal symptoms nor any fevers and there has been some improvement with paracetamol.

Toby has become increasingly clumsy and has had several unexpected falls even when sitting. Having walked up stairs independently, he now wants to hold the rail or someone's hand and no longer runs with confidence. He has fallen off his tricycle twice and no longer wants to ride it.

Toby is the youngest of three children and has no significant past medical or family history. He had chickenpox 3 years ago. Up to now his development has been normal and he is fully immunized.

Examination

Toby appears a generally healthy boy with his height and weight on the 25th centiles and his head circumference on the 50th centile. There is no cervical lymphadenopathy and passive movements of his neck are normal, although he is reluctant to look up to the ceiling. His pulse is 88 beats/min and his blood pressure is 85/60 mmHg. There are no murmurs, and examination of the respiratory and abdominal systems is unremarkable. There are no neurocutaneous markers. There is no nystagmus and external ocular movements are normal. Fundoscopy is very difficult because he screws up his eyes, but a brief glimpse of the right fundus suggests blurred disc margins. The remainder of the cranial nerves appear normal. He has a broad-based, unsteady gait and cannot walk heel to toe. However, muscle bulk, tone, power and reflexes are normal in both arms and legs. He is very unsteady when standing with his eyes shut. He tries very hard with the finger–nose test but misses both every time, nor can he touch his nose accurately with his eyes shut. He can pick up small objects without a problem.

Questions
- What movement disorder do these symptoms and signs describe?
- Where is the pathology likely to be located and what complication has arisen?
- What investigation does he need?

ANSWER 52

Toby has symptoms and signs of ataxia – the inability to make smooth, accurate and coordinated movements. Observation during play is the key to much of the neurological examination in a child. It is crucial to take account of the developmental stage of the child – a broad-based, unsteady gait is normal for a child who is just starting to walk but not in a previously confident 4-year-old. Other tests of ataxia include the heel–shin test and dysdiadochokinesia, but he is probably too young for these to be interpretable. Make these formal parts fun and most children will very happily do their best. Remember that, by definition, all tests for movement disorders require the ability to move; hence tone and power must be assessed. Similarly he must be able to see to do the coordination tests.

Ataxia is usually due to disorders of the cerebellum and/or the sensory pathways in the posterior columns of the spinal cord. The neck pain, rubbing of his head in distress and vomiting are highly suggestive of raised intracranial pressure (ICP). Unfortunately, this is frequently missed in children because they are poor at localizing pain and the symptoms are relatively non-specific and common. Fundoscopy is notoriously difficult in children because they don't cooperate and you may only get the briefest glimpse. Hypertension and bradycardia are usually late signs when the child is obtunded. The classic early morning headache and effortless vomiting of adults with raised ICP is less common in children.

The cerebellum is therefore the most likely location for the pathology, with the raised ICP being due to hydrocephalus secondary to obstruction of the fourth ventricle. It could be due to a congenital anomaly of the cerebellum, such as the Dandy–Walker syndrome or a Chiari malformation, but his symptoms are relatively recent. Vomiting is a major feature of acute cerebellar ataxia following a viral illness such as chickenpox, but the onset is sudden and often severe with nystagmus and dysarthria and the other symptoms and signs of raised ICP are often absent. A space-occupying lesion is most likely in our case.

In children, two-thirds of brain tumours are located in the posterior fossa compared with one-third in adults. Toby needs an urgent MRI (or CT) scan.

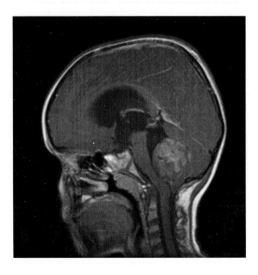

Figure 52.1 Sagittal MRI scan of Toby's brain.

The MRI scan (Fig. 52.1) shows a vermian midline posterior fossa tumour with hydrocephalus. At posterior craniotomy, as much tumour as possible was resected and the hydrocephalus resolved without him needing a ventriculoperitoneal shunt. Histology confirmed a medulloblastoma, a primitive neuroectodermal tumour (PNET), which is the most common malignant brain tumour of childhood. Medulloblastomas frequently spread through the leptomeninges and patients require cerebrospinal fluid analysis. Treatment recognizes this risk and usually includes craniospinal irradiation. In recent years prognosis has improved to 70–80 per cent with the introduction of additional intensive systemic chemotherapy.

KEY POINTS

- Raised intracranial pressure in children frequently presents with non-specific symptoms.
- Two-thirds of childhood brain tumours are located in the posterior fossa.

History

Munira is a 7-year-old Asian girl who presents to the paediatric rapid referral clinic with a lump on the side of her neck. Her mother noticed it a week earlier. It is not painful. She has had no fevers, night sweats or weight loss. Her mother states that, about 4 weeks ago, she had a cold that lasted for 2 days and was not accompanied by a temperature. Munira had the BCG vaccine when she was a baby. There is no family history or history of contact with TB. There has been no travel in the last 6 months.

Examination

Munira is apyrexial. There is a 4 × 3 cm lump on the left side of the neck. It is not erythematous, warm or tender. It is mobile and not attached to the skin. There are some small (<1 cm) lymph nodes on the right side of the neck. There is no lymphadenopathy elsewhere and no hepatosplenomegaly. A BCG scar is seen. The ear, nose and throat appear normal and there are no signs in the other systems. The child is investigated and reviewed 48 hours later with the results.

INVESTIGATIONS		
		Normal
Haemoglobin	10.7 g/dL	10.5–13.5 g/dL
White cell count	10.3×10^9/L	$4.0–11.0 \times 10^9$/L
Neutrophils	7.2×10^9/L	$1.7–7.5 \times 10^9$/L
Platelets	430×10^9/L	$150–400 \times 10^9$/L
C-reactive protein (CRP)	12 mg/L	<6 mg/L
Erythrocyte sedimentation rate (ESR)	24 mm/hr	0–15 mm/hr
Anti-streptolysin O titre (ASOT)	<200 IU/ml	<200 IU/ml
Paul–Bunnell test	Negative	
Chest X-ray	Normal	

Neck ultrasound – several enlarged lymph nodes seen, the largest 2.2 cm in diameter. No fluid collection seen

Mantoux test (read at 48 hours) – negative

Questions

- What is the differential diagnosis at presentation (prior to the investigation results)?
- Would you administer any treatment at the first visit?
- What is the most likely diagnosis following the investigation results?
- What course of action would you follow if there was no change in the size of the lump after 10 days?

ANSWER 53

The lump is consistent with enlarged lymph nodes. The differential diagnosis is:

- infection – bacterial, viral or mycobacteria (tuberculosis and non-tuberculous mycobacteria)
- malignancy – lymphoma or leukaemia.

Lymph nodes are often palpable in children. Cervical and axillary lymph nodes >1 cm in diameter and inguinal lymph nodes >1.5 cm in diameter are considered to be enlarged. Any enlargement in any other lymph nodes, e.g. supraclavicular, requires further investigation. All children get several upper respiratory tract infections a year, and the minor cold several weeks earlier is probably irrelevant. Statistically, a bacterial cervical lymphadenitis is the most likely diagnosis. However, usually there is a clear history of a current or recent upper respiratory tract infection. In bacterial infections, the overlying skin is usually erythematous and the lump is warm and tender. Occasionally the swelling may become fluctuant and this is indicative of pus formation and an abscess. In such a case, a referral should be made to a surgeon for incision and drainage. In viral infections, the nodes are tender but are not usually warm or erythematous. The Paul–Bunnell test is similar to the Monospot test and is a test for glandular fever. Viral serology for HIV, cytomegalovirus, toxoplasmosis (which often produce more generalized lymphadenopathy) and cat scratch disease (due to *Bartonella henselae*) would be helpful if there was still no diagnosis after the initial investigations.

In tuberculosis, the lump is cold and non-tender. Munira has had her BCG vaccination but it is important to remember that, although this vaccination provides reasonable protection against miliary TB and TB meningitis (50–80 per cent), it only provides 50 per cent protection for pulmonary TB and only minimal (if any) protection against non-tuberculous mycobacteria. A lymphoma can present with non-tender cervical lymphadenopathy. The lymph nodes tend to be firmer than inflammatory nodes and may be adherent to the overlying skin or underlying structures. The absence of systemic symptoms, such as fevers, night sweats and weight loss, makes the diagnosis of tuberculosis and lymphoma less likely.

At the first visit, it would be worth giving a 10-day course of an antibiotic, e.g. co-amoxiclav, that would treat streptococcal and staphylococcal infection. This would treat the most likely diagnosis of a bacterial lymphadenitis.

The white blood cell count is normal and the CRP and ESR are only mildly elevated. The ASOT, Paul–Bunnell test and Mantoux are negative. These results make an infection unlikely and a malignancy the most likely diagnosis.

If there was no diminution in the size of the lump following the 10-day course of treatment (which would suggest that the diagnosis is not a bacterial lymphadenitis), the patient should be referred to a surgeon for an urgent biopsy. This was the case with Munira in whom the lymph node biopsy was diagnostic of Hodgkin's lymphoma.

 KEY POINTS

- Most children have some small palpable lymph nodes.
- The commonest cause of cervical lymphadenitis is streptococcal or staphylococcal infection.
- Patients with lymphoma commonly present with non-tender firm cervical lymphadenopathy.

CASE 54: A SWOLLEN SHOULDER

History

Naomi is a 13-year-old girl who presents to the A&E department of her local hospital for the third time in 8 weeks. On the first occasion she had slipped from her horse whilst mounting and sustained some minor bruising mainly to the right arm, hip and leg. There was no evidence of any serious bone injury. Over the course of the next 2 weeks she developed worsening pain and immobility in her right shoulder. Examination from that visit was recorded as showing a decreased range of movement but little else. Her symptoms were thought to be due to either a 'frozen shoulder' or to be functional, and she was prescribed ibuprofen for pain and referred for routine physiotherapy. The physiotherapists have sent her back with increasing pain and now swelling.

Examination

Naomi is clearly in pain and is reluctant to move her right shoulder. There is a generalized, smooth, warm, firm swelling of the right shoulder with a decreased range of movement in all directions. There are some distended visible veins and the overlying skin is shiny but not red. The remainder of the examination is normal.

INVESTIGATIONS
Naomi's shoulder X-ray is shown in Figure 54.1.

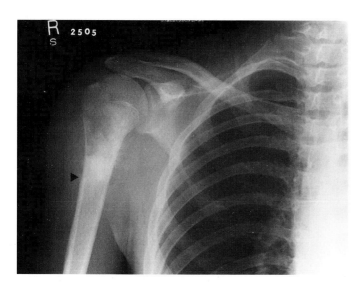

Figure 54.1 Naomi's shoulder X-ray.

Questions
- What is the diagnosis?
- What is the management?

ANSWER 54

The diagnosis is an osteosarcoma of the right humerus. There is no differential. This is a malignant tumour that classically presents in adolescence and often comes to light after a relatively minor injury. It is still not uncommon for there to be a delay in diagnosis because it is rare and not considered in the differential diagnosis of limb and joint pain. The characteristic features on the X-ray are:

- bone destruction
- gross swelling
- elevation of the periosteum with creation of Codman's triangle (marked with an arrow ▶ on the X-ray)
- 'sunray' spicules of new bone visible in the muscle and subcutaneous tissues.

The first step is regular adequate pain relief. Non-steroidal anti-inflammatory agents may be adequate but it is highly likely that opioids will be needed. This is an aggressive tumour with rapid expansion of the periosteum which is exquisitely painful.

Secondly, a senior paediatrician – preferably from the local 'shared care' oncology team – should break the news to the girl and her family. They will be devastated and quite possibly angry at the perceived delay in diagnosis. The local team will have the experience and knowledge to answer any immediate questions. They will also know that the best route for onward referral is to a specialist paediatric oncology centre and not, at this stage, to orthopaedics. Although a tissue diagnosis is required, she needs to be screened for metastases as this may alter the management significantly. Osteosarcomas usually spread to lung and bone and she will need a chest CT scan and a bone scan plus an MRI scan of the shoulder to guide future surgery. The biopsy should only be taken in a specialist centre (or with their explicit agreement) and reviewed by a team of specialist histopathologists.

The specific management of osteosarcoma is initial chemotherapy to reduce tumour bulk and to clear any metastases, followed by surgery followed by further chemotherapy. Definitive surgery is probably contraindicated if metastases have not cleared or significantly reduced with initial chemotherapy, although some patients with isolated lung secondaries do extremely well following their resection. Modern surgery is largely successful at avoiding mutilating amputation using prostheses that can be externally 'lengthened' as the patient grows.

Prognosis depends upon the presence of metastatic spread at presentation – bone secondaries carry a particularly grave outlook – and on response to chemotherapy as evidenced by tumour necrosis at surgical resection. More than 90 per cent necrosis is associated with an improved outcome. Overall prognosis is a 5-year survival rate of approximately 60 per cent.

 KEY POINTS

- Children do not get 'frozen shoulder' and functional pain is a diagnosis of exclusion.
- Bone tumours are rare but should be considered in any patient with unexpectedly severe symptoms following a minor injury.
- The care of children with cancer should be coordinated by a specialist centre.
- Centralization of care, entry into randomized controlled trials and the use of national or international protocols have steadily improved the prognosis in childhood cancer.

History

The parents of 6-year-old Lucy, who has B-cell lymphoma, have brought her to the children's ward of their local hospital as they have recorded a temperature at home of 38.7°C. They have since given her a dose of paracetamol. Lucy completed her second course of chemotherapy 6 days previously. They know that her last blood count 2 days ago showed that she was neutropenic (neutrophils <1.0 × 10⁹/L). The whole family, including the patient, have had symptoms of a viral illness with a sore throat, a runny nose and a bit of a cough, but she has also had three bouts of diarrhoea in the preceding 24 hours and some lower abdominal pain. There are four other children at home, ranging in age from 6 months to 9 years. The mother works part-time in the evenings serving behind a bar, while the father is a self-employed painter and decorator. Their daughter was very sick at presentation and spent 5 weeks in the regional paediatric oncology centre 40 miles away. She has only been home since the end of the recent course of chemotherapy.

Examination

Lucy is playing in a side-room with her dolls. She is reluctant to be examined. Her temperature is 37.4°C. Her pulse is 130 beats/min and her blood pressure 95/60 mmHg. Oxygen saturation is 97 per cent in air. The indwelling central-line exit site is slightly erythematous and tender. There are no murmurs and examination of the respiratory and abdominal systems is unremarkable. Her ears, nose and throat are normal.

INVESTIGATIONS		
		Normal
Haemoglobin	7.4 g/dL	11.5–15.5 g/dL
White cell count	0.6 × 10⁹/L	6.0–17.5 × 10⁹/L
Neutrophils	0.1 × 10⁹/L	3.0–5.8 × 10⁹/L
Platelets	24 × 10⁹/L	150–400 × 10⁹/L
Sodium	134 mmol/L	138–146 mmol/L
Potassium	3.8 mmol/L	3.5–5.0 mmol/L
Urea	6.2 mmol/L	1.8–6.4 mmol/L
Creatinine	64 µmol/L	27–62 µmol/L
C-reactive protein	67 mg/L	<6 mg/L

Questions

- What factors increase the risk of infection in children with cancer?
- What is the management?

ANSWER 55

Once a child with cancer undergoing treatment is in remission, the commonest cause of death is infection. Families have written instructions about temperature monitoring and when to seek advice. All admitting hospitals have protocols for treatment based on the degree of fever (e.g. $\geqslant 38.5°C$) and the neutrophil count (e.g. $<0.75 \times 10^9/L$).

> **!** **Contributing factors to infection in children with cancer**
>
> - Neutropenia – the more severe ($<0.5 \times 109/L$) and prolonged, the greater the risk. There may be loss of the inflammatory response, e.g. insufficient white blood cells to form an abscess
> - Mucositis – following radiotherapy or chemotherapy. Can affect the whole gastrointestinal tract. There is a risk that intestinal bacteria will breach the gut wall and enter the bloodstream
> - Indwelling central lines – crucial for giving chemotherapy and blood sampling, but significant source of infection, both blood-borne and at exit site
> - Frequent hospital admissions
> - Poor nutrition
> - Generalized immunosuppression, inhibiting the usual host defences – viruses that rarely cause severe illness in immunocompetent children can be life-threatening in oncology patients, e.g. varicella, measles and cytomegalovirus. Chemotherapy also predisposes children to 'opportunistic infections' – organisms that only infect an immunocompromised host. Prophylaxis against *Pneumocystis carinii* is included in protocols for cancers where the chemotherapy regimen is particularly immunosuppressive

---

The reduction in temperature is irrelevant – the protocols are initiated on the recorded temperature at home. That she is playing is also irrelevant – she has worrying symptoms and signs. Abdominal pain and diarrhoea suggest mucositis and she is tachycardic. Although a visible source of sepsis is her central line site, this rarely causes significant systemic features. Gram-negative sepsis is the real threat and she requires admission and the immediate administration of intravenous broad-spectrum antibiotics that include cover for Gram-negative bacteria (e.g. *Pseudomonas aeruginosa*, *Klebsiella*), as well as Gram-positive bacteria that may be causing a line infection.

Blood cultures and swabs (e.g. throat and line site) must be taken first and preferably urine and stool samples. However, collecting these should never delay antibiotics. A chest X-ray is needed if there are respiratory symptoms or signs. Careful monitoring and frequent re-evaluation are required, changing the regimen according to response and culture results, e.g. coagulase-negative staphylococci frequently cause infections in central lines. If Lucy is still febrile and significantly neutropenic after about 5 days, antifungal agents may be added. Haemopoietic growth factors, e.g. granulocyte colony-stimulating factor, are sometimes given. She will almost certainly need blood and/or platelet transfusions. Again, protocols vary but an example would be a haemoglobin $<7\,g/dL$ and platelets $<10 \times 10^9/L$ or active bleeding.

Once afebrile and recovering, she can be discharged home where, if necessary, the parents or community nurses can continue antibiotics. Life for such families is inevitably disrupted socially and financially – the main breadwinner here is self-employed. They will be supported by specific staff and charities.

 KEY POINTS

- Once in remission, infection is the commonest cause of death in children receiving treatment for cancer.
- Febrile neutropenia in an immunocompromised child is a medical emergency.
- Common viral illnesses can kill immunocompromised children.

History
Hannah is a 5-year-old girl seen in the paediatric day unit at the request of the GP. Hannah has been seen several times in the past few weeks with non-specific symptoms. Initially she was just off-colour and lacking in energy, wanting to sit and watch television rather than play outside. She was complaining that her legs were aching and she needed regular doses of paracetamol. The GP and her parents thought this might all be related to her recently starting full-time school and her mother went in to talk to the staff, worried about possible bullying. Hannah then had an ear infection with a high temperature that was slow to respond to antibiotics and was therefore assumed to be viral. Her admission has been precipitated this week because she has started to refuse to walk, complaining that 'she hurts all over'. The GP requested a full blood count (FBC) and erythrocyte sedimentation rate (ESR) and has been phoned with the results below.

Examination
Hannah is quiet and pale. She is sitting on her mother's knee and is reluctant to be examined, crying when she is moved. Her temperature is 37.8°C. She has widespread lymphadenopathy, including supraclavicular. She is clinically anaemic but not jaundiced. She has bruises on her shins, left thigh and right upper arm. Her pulse is 96 beats/min and heart sounds are normal, but she has a grade 2 systolic murmur located at the left sternal edge. Her chest is clear. In the abdomen there is 4 cm hepatomegaly and her spleen is palpable 2 cm below the left costal margin. Her left ear drum is dull and pink but the right is normal, as is her throat. Although she resists movement of her joints, there is no obvious swelling, deformity or overlying skin change.

🔍 INVESTIGATIONS		
		Normal
Haemoglobin	7.3 g/dL	11.5–15.5 g/dL
White cell count	3.4×10^9/L	$5.5–15.5 \times 10^9$/L
Neutrophils	1.3×10^9/L	$3.0–5.8 \times 10^9$/L
Lymphocytes	1.8×10^9/L	$1.5–3.0 \times 10^9$/L
Platelets	36×10^9/L	$150–400 \times 10^9$/L
ESR	88 mm/hour	0–10 mm/hour
Blood film	Atypical lymphocytes seen	

Questions
- What is the most likely diagnosis?
- How can it be confirmed?
- Outline the treatment of this condition
- What factors are associated with a poor prognosis?

ANSWER 56

Hannah's blood count shows pancytopenia, which is due to either bone marrow (BM) infiltration or failure (see Case **48**, A pale child, p. 143). She has the clinical symptoms and signs of infiltration – the bone pain is due to marrow expansion. Children may not localize the pain, and generalized non-specific symptoms culminating in a reluctance to move and weight-bear are common. There may be bone tenderness. Hannah has evidence of extramedullary involvement with hepatosplenomegaly and lymphadenopathy. Supraclavicular nodes are always suspicious. Bruises below the knees are very common in children, but those at sites other than the shins may be pathological. The murmur is almost certainly a flow murmur due to anaemia. The most likely diagnosis is acute leukaemia, probably lymphoblastic (ALL) because this accounts for 80 per cent of leukaemias in childhood.

Leukaemic 'blast' cells may not be observed on a routine peripheral blood film examination or may be misinterpreted. The peripheral FBC may even be normal, causing diagnostic difficulty in differentiating it from conditions that present with similar features, e.g. infectious mononucleosis or rheumatoid arthritis. Analysis of a BM aspirate is essential. This differentiates ALL from acute myeloid leukaemia (AML) and other malignant causes of BM infiltration, such as neuroblastoma. It also enables classification of ALL using cell membrane markers and cytogenetic and molecular genetic features which influence treatment decisions and prognosis.

Current treatment for ALL is in four phases:

1. *Remission induction.* Four weeks of combination chemotherapy. More than 95 per cent show BM remission by day 28.
2. *Consolidation and CNS protection.* Oral chemotherapy is commenced. Cytotoxic drugs penetrate poorly into the CNS. A course of weekly intrathecal (IT) drugs is given to prevent later CNS relapse. IT drugs are also given during induction and throughout maintenance.
3. *Delayed intensification(s).* Remission at day 28 is often only apparent. One or two courses (depending on risk) of intense chemotherapy are dovetailed with blocks of maintenance chemotherapy.
4. *Continuing maintenance.* Chemotherapy continues for a total of 2 years in girls and 3 years in boys. Patients are immunosuppressed and at risk of opportunistic infections. Co-trimoxazole is given to prevent *Pneumocystis carinii* pneumonia.

! **Poor prognostic factors in acute lymphoblastic leukaemia**

- Total white cell count $>100 \times 10^9$/L at presentation
- Outside age range 2–10 years
- Male sex
- T-cell (15 per cent) or mature B-cell (1 per cent) origin (Common-ALL (85 per cent) from B-cell progenitors has best prognosis)
- Certain chromosome abnormalities – hypodiploidy, presence of Philadelphia chromosome (Others, e.g. hyperdiploidy, confer a favourable prognosis)
- CNS disease at presentation
- Slow response to treatment, >5% blasts persisting on day 28 BM

Overall prognosis for ALL is excellent with a 5-year survival >80 per cent.

KEY POINTS

- Acute leukaemia can present with very non-specific and indolent clinical features.
- A bone marrow aspirate is essential to confirm or refute a diagnosis of acute leukaemia.

BONES AND JOINTS

CASE 57: A GIRL WITH A LIMP

History

Janis is a 12-year-old girl who presents to the paediatric rapid referral clinic with a 4-month history of an intermittent pain in her left hip with an associated limp. The pain is worse on running and she has stopped participating in her physical education classes at school. She occasionally takes ibuprofen that provides some pain relief. There is no history of trauma. She is generally well. She had a tonsillectomy and adenoidectomy at 5 years of age. Her mother has hypothyroidism.

Examination

She is apyrexial. She has an obvious limp. The left hip is flexed and there is restriction of internal rotation, abduction and flexion. There are no signs in the left knee or foot and there are no other joint abnormalities. The back is normal. There are no abdominal signs and no neurological signs in the lower limbs.

Janis's weight, at 55.4 kg, is between the 91st and 98th centiles and her height, at 1.34 m, is just below the second centile.

INVESTIGATIONS		
		Normal
Haemoglobin	10.8 g/dL	10.5–13.5 g/dL
White cell count	8.3×10^9/L	$4.0–11.0 \times 10^9$/L
Neutrophils	5.2×10^9/L	$1.7–7.5 \times 10^9$/L
Platelets	230×10^9/L	$150–400 \times 10^9$/L
C-reactive protein	4 mg/L	<6 mg/L
Erythrocyte sedimentation rate	14 mm/hour	0–15 mm/hour
Anteroposterior X-ray of the pelvis and hips – normal		

Janis's lateral hip X-ray is shown in Figure 57.1.

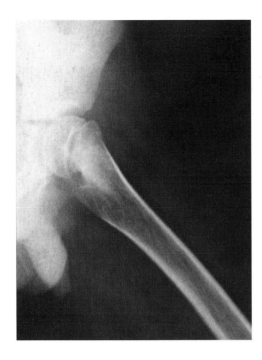

Figure 57.1 Janis's lateral hip X-ray.
(Reproduced with permission from McRae
R, *Clinical Orthopaedic Examination*, 2003,
Churchill Livingstone.)

Questions

- What are the common causes of a limp in a child?
- What is the diagnosis?
- What further investigations should be done?
- What is the treatment?

ANSWER 57

A limp is a common problem in childhood. It is important to be aware that it can be due to an abnormality anywhere from the back to the foot.

Causes of a limp in a child are best considered according to age:

- *0–3 years*
  - Trauma, e.g. fracture (may be accidental or non-accidental)
  - Infection: septic arthritis, osteomyelitis or discitis
  - Malignancy
  - Developmental dysplasia of the hip
  - Neuromuscular disease, e.g. cerebral palsy
- *4–10 years*
  - Trauma
  - Transient synovitis (irritable hip)
  - Infection – septic arthritis, osteomyelitis or discitis
  - Perthe's disease
  - Juvenile idiopathic arthritis
  - Malignancy, e.g. leukaemia
  - Neuromuscular disease, e.g. cerebral palsy
- *10–18 years*
  - Trauma
  - Infection: septic arthritis, osteomyelitis or discitis
  - Slipped upper femoral epiphysis
  - Juvenile idiopathic arthritis
  - Malignancy, e.g. osteogenic sarcoma

The diagnosis is a slipped upper femoral epiphysis (SUFE). SUFE is commoner in boys and in obese individuals. Pain can be felt in the groin, hip or thigh or there may be referred pain in the knee. Classically the affected hip is flexed and the leg is externally rotated. A small slip may be missed on the anteroposterior view and a lateral or frog leg view of the hip is therefore also necessary. The lateral X-ray shows displacement of the proximal femoral epiphysis relative to the femoral neck. Approximately 25 per cent of patients will also have a contralateral slip and the other hip must therefore be carefully assessed.

A minority of patients with SUFE have an underlying endocrinopathy or metabolic abnormality (hypothyroidism, hypogonadism, growth hormone abnormalities, panhypo-pituitarism or renal osteodystrophy) and if this is suspected then the appropriate investigations should be performed. Janis is short and overweight and has a family history of thyroid disease. A more detailed examination demonstrated that she had a small goitre. Thyroid function tests revealed a free T4 of 9.2 pmol/L (12–22), a thyroid-stimulating hormone (TSH) of 64 mU/L (0.5–6.0) and thyroid peroxidase (TPO) antibodies of 1342 IU/mL (0–34). These results are compatible with a diagnosis of Hashimoto's (autoimmune) thyroiditis. Obese individuals should have their fasting glucose measured and this test should also be done on Janis.

Janis should be admitted and told not to weight-bear. She should be referred urgently to the orthopaedic surgeons. Although it would seem that the SUFE has been present for 4 months, one can get an acute or chronic slip of the epiphysis that can lead to avascular necrosis of the femoral head. Surgery is therefore urgent and consists of pinning the femoral head to the femoral neck. Thyroxine should also be started.

KEY POINTS
<ul><li>In SUFE, a lateral or frog leg view, as well as an anteroposterior view, of the hip is necessary to avoid missing minor slips.</li><li>Urgent treatment is necessary in SUFE to try to avoid the complication of avascular necrosis of the femoral head</li></ul>

History

Kyle is a 16-month-old boy who presents to the paediatric day unit with a 2-day history of intermittent inconsolable crying and fevers up to 40°C. He has not been interested in food and has vomited twice. There has been no diarrhoea. His parents report that he seems to be in pain when his nappy is changed. He had a cut on his right foot 2 weeks ago which has healed and there is no obvious history of trauma. Kyle was born at term and has no other significant past medical history. Both parents are unemployed and he has two older half-sisters, aged 5 and 3, with the same mother. He is on no regular medication and has no known allergies.

Examination

He looks unwell with a temperature of 38.7°C. He dislikes handling and is clearly in pain. His capillary refill time is 4 s and he is mildly dehydrated. His pulse is 135 beats/min and his blood pressure is 75/50 mmHg. There is no skin rash. Examination of the cardiovascular and respiratory systems is unremarkable. His abdomen seems soft with no obvious tenderness or organomegaly. Bowel sounds are normal. There is no meningism. Examination of the ears, nose and throat is normal.

INVESTIGATIONS		
		Normal
Haemoglobin	12.3 g/dL	11.5–15.5 g/dL
White cell count (WCC)	28.0 × 10⁹/L	6.0–17.5 × 10⁹/L
Neutrophils	22.0 × 10⁹/L	3.0–5.8 × 10⁹/L
Platelets	325 × 10⁹/L	150–400 × 10⁹/L
Erythrocyte sedimentation rate (ESR)	78 mm/hour	0–10 mm/hour
Sodium	140 mmol/L	138–146 mmol/L
Potassium	4.5 mmol/L	3.5–5.0 mmol/L
Urea	3.7 mmol/L	1.8–6.4 mmol/L
Creatinine	46 μmol/L	27–62 μmol/L
C-reactive protein (CRP)	340 mg/L	<6 mg/L
Urine microscopy	No abnormality detected	
Lumbar puncture	No white blood cells, no organisms seen	
Chest X-ray	Clear	

Questions

- What else should you document in the examination?
- What is the most likely diagnosis?
- What imaging modalities would you consider?
- What is the management?

ANSWER 58

This boy has signs of sepsis with fever, prolonged capillary refill time and tachycardia. His investigations support this. The history of pain with movement is strongly suggestive of musculoskeletal pathology. In acute sepsis, the emphasis is usually on diagnosing meningitis or an acute abdomen and it is easy to overlook this system. Examine for any swelling, redness of the skin, warmth and tenderness. There may be nothing to see superficially, so observe the posture and whether the child is keeping any limb flexed or still. Gently examine the range of movement of all joints.

The most likely diagnosis is osteomyelitis or septic arthritis. The legs are much the commonest site and most infections are blood-borne. There is often a recent history of minor trauma or a breach in the skin, which probably explains why boys are more often affected. The commonest bacteria involved is *Staphylococcus aureus*.

Children with sickle cell disease have a higher incidence of skeletal infections. The differential depends on the site but includes soft-tissue infections and psoas abscess. In the less obviously septic child, remember trauma, both accidental and non-accidental, and bone infiltration with cancers such as leukaemia.

! | **Possible imaging modalities**

- Plain X-rays – excludes trauma. In osteomyelitis, bones are unlikely to be abnormal until 10–14 days after onset. In arthritis they are often normal but may show widening of joint space ± local soft tissue or fat changes
- Ultrasound (US) – highly sensitive in detecting joint effusion and guiding aspiration. It may demonstrate swelling and distortion of soft tissues and subperiosteal region
- MRI – the best technique to differentiate between soft tissue and bone infection; also to detect a joint effusion where US is normal. However, the boy will need sedation or general anaesthetic at this age
- Technetium (^{99m}Tc) bone scan – accumulates as 'hot spots' in areas of increased bone turnover so useful in osteomyelitis, especially multifocal. Infection close to growth plates can limit specificity

---

First, he needs fluid resuscitation and adequate pain relief. If the clinical diagnosis is osteomyelitis, he should start intravenous antibiotics, e.g. co-amoxiclav. However, if there is evidence of septic arthritis, he should ideally have an immediate US and, if there is an effusion, an urgent arthrotomy before starting antibiotics. If there is no effusion, the diagnosis is more likely to be osteomyelitis and antibiotics can be started. They should not be delayed in order to establish a definitive diagnosis with imaging or cultures, because this increases the risk of long-term effects on the growth and function of the affected limb, especially if the growth plate is involved. The length of treatment and route of administration of antibiotics for both depend upon the clinical and biochemical (WCC, ESR, CRP) responses. A total of 6 weeks is common practice. Long-term follow-up is necessary because problems may not be apparent for several years. Most children make an uneventful recovery.

 KEY POINTS

- Bone and/or joint sepsis should be considered in the differential diagnosis of all children presenting with sepsis.
- Delay in treatment of osteomyelitis or septic arthritis can cause significant long-term effects on the growth and function of the affected limb.

CASE 59: SWOLLEN JOINTS

History

Zoe is a 3-year-old girl referred to children's outpatients. For the past 7 weeks she has been generally off-colour and miserable. Having loved nursery she is increasingly reluctant to get up in the morning and is taking ages to get dressed. She says she feels 'stiff all over'. As the day goes by, her stiffness improves unless she has been sitting for a while, but she is still easily tired and lacks energy. When encouraged to walk, she does so very slowly and wants to be carried or use the buggy. Zoe has also been complaining that her knees and ankles hurt and her parents report intermittent but definite swelling of her left knee and right ankle. Her symptoms are helped by ibuprofen. There are no reports of injury. She had a sore throat 2 months ago but has not had any fevers since, or any rashes. Zoe has no significant past medical or family history. She has a healthy 9-month-old brother.

Examination

Zoe is a quiet but generally healthy girl sitting on her mother's knee. She would not walk into the consulting room. Her height is on the 75th centile and her weight is on the 50th. She is not clinically anaemic or clubbed and there is no lymphadenopathy. She is afebrile. There are no rashes. Both knees and her right ankle are mildly swollen and feel warm to touch, but there is no overlying skin change. The left knee seems most affected. There is pain and a decreased range of movement. There are similar findings in the proximal interphalangeal joint of the left index finger. The remainder of her joints, including the hips, appear normal. Examination of the cardiovascular, respiratory and abdominal systems is normal with no hepatosplenomegaly.

INVESTIGATIONS		
		Normal
Haemoglobin	11.8 g/dL	11.5–15.5 g/dL
White cell count	9.2×10^9/L	$6.0–17.5 \times 10^9$/L
Platelets	395×10^9/L	$150–400 \times 10^9$/L
Erythrocyte sedimentation rate (ESR)	19 mm/hour	0–10 mm/hr
Urea and electrolytes	Normal	
Liver function tests	Normal	
Bone chemistry	Normal	
C-reactive protein (CRP)	21 mg/L	<6 mg/L
Anti-nuclear antibody (ANA)	Mildly positive	Negative
Rheumatoid factor	Negative	Negative

Questions

- What is the differential diagnosis?
- Which of these is most likely?
- What else needs to be formally examined?
- What are the principles of management?

ANSWER 59

Zoe has a polyarthritis – pain, swelling, warmth and restricted movement of several joints. The much commoner arthralgia is joint pain without the other features.

! **Differential diagnosis of chronic polyarthritis**

- Connective tissue disorder – juvenile idiopathic arthritis (JIA), systemic lupus erythematosus, dermatomyositis, psoriatic arthritis
- Infection – bacterial causes are unlikely with this chronic history. Viruses such as hepatitis and also Lyme disease should be excluded
- Malignant disorders – children with leukaemia can have joint pain due to metaphyseal marrow expansion months before peripheral blood count changes. A bone marrow examination may be indicated
- Inflammatory bowel disease – can present with arthritis
- Vasculitis – Henoch–Schönlein purpura

Zoe has other features in the history that make JIA the most likely diagnosis. There has been an insidious onset of early morning stiffness, 'gelling' (stiffness) after inactivity, slow walking and progressive joint involvement. Juvenile idiopathic arthritis is a group of conditions in which there is a chronic arthritis lasting >6 consecutive weeks before the age of 16 years. Infection and other causes must obviously be excluded. Her sore throat 2 months earlier is probably incidental although a reactive arthritis following *Streptococcus* tonsillitis is well recognized and the anti-streptolysin O titre (ASOT) should be assayed. Juvenile idiopathic arthritis is classified according to its onset as systemic, polyarticular (> four joints) or oligo(pauci)articular (≤ four joints).

Zoe has oligoarticular JIA, the commonest subtype, which typically affects the knees and ankles and less often the elbows or a single finger joint in young children <6 years, particularly girls. In systemic or polyarticular JIA, there is often laboratory evidence of chronic inflammation with anaemia, thrombocytosis and an elevated ESR and C-reactive protein, but in oligoarticular JIA these may be normal or only mildly abnormal. Patients with oligoarticular JIA have an increased risk of one of the complications of JIA, chronic anterior uveitis, and this is increased still further in girls who are ANA-positive. She therefore needs formal ophthalmology screening and frequent regular review. The course of the uveitis is independent of the joints.

! **Principles of management**

- Pain control with non-steroidal anti-inflammatory drugs (NSAIDs)
- Physiotherapy, hydrotherapy and occupational therapy. Splints may help prevent contractures and deformities
- Intra-articular depot corticosteroid injections to reduce swelling and deformity
- Disease-modifying drugs are needed if not controlled with NSAIDs, e.g. methotrexate, sulphasalazine. Cytokine inhibitors (e.g. anti-tumour necrosis factor) may be needed for refractory polyarticular or systemic JIA. All of these need careful monitoring in a specialist setting
- Regular monitoring of growth and nutrition as for any chronic disease
- Multidisciplinary team approach, including psychosocial support. The impact of all forms of JIA is significant, although the prognosis for oligoarthritis is generally better than for other groups

---

	KEY POINTS

- Juvenile idiopathic arthritis can only be diagnosed after 6 continuous weeks of arthritis and after the exclusion of other causes.
- The management of JIA requires a multidisciplinary team with as much emphasis on the therapies as on drug interventions.

History

Melissa is a 12-year-old who presents to her GP with a persistent cough that has been going on for 3 weeks. The whole family have had a flu-like illness but her symptoms seem to have gone on for longer. Her cough is non-productive, she has not been short of breath and she hasn't complained of chest pain. She had a temperature early on but this has resolved. There is no significant past medical history and she rarely attends the surgery. She has not yet started her periods. She takes no regular medication.

Examination

Melissa is a generally healthy girl who is not distressed at rest. She is pink in room air and not clubbed. There is no significant lymphadenopathy. The GP examines her respiratory system and can find no abnormalities. However, he notices that she appears to have a lateral curvature to the left of her thoracic spine. There are no neurocutaneous features.

Questions
- What is this deformity?
- What else should now be documented in the history and examination?
- What are the management options?

ANSWER 60

This patient has a abnormality in spinal alignment in the coronal plane – a scoliosis. The spine has normal curves in the sagittal plane that provide stability and balance. The cervical and lumbar spines are convex anteriorly, termed lordosis. The thoracic and sacral spines are convex posteriorly, termed kyphosis. These normal curves can be exaggerated, e.g. in congenital deformities such as achondroplasia where there is almost always a significant lumbar lordosis.

Having found a scoliosis, the next question is whether it is postural (common) or structural (rare). A postural scoliosis may be caused by pain or be secondary to a leg-length discrepancy and these conditions should be ruled out first. Leg-length discrepancy is usually easily managed with a shoe raise. Provided both are absent, a postural scoliosis will disappear when the child bends forwards to try to touch her toes and no further intervention is required. In a structural scoliosis, the curvature persists in the forward-bending test and there is rotation of the vertebral bodies towards the convexity of the curve, causing a 'rib hump'. Most cases of structural scoliosis are idiopathic but some are related to an underlying condition and these need exclusion.

! **Differential diagnosis of a structural scoliosis**

- Idiopathic
- Neuromuscular, e.g. cerebral palsy or Duchenne muscular dystrophy
- Congenital structural abnormalities of the vertebrae, e.g. hemivertebrae – there is a high risk of associated spinal cord defects, e.g. spinal dysraphism and other congenital abnormalities, especially genitourinary
- Syndromic, e.g. neurofibromatosis and Marfan syndrome

Therefore, children with a structural scoliosis need a thorough neurological evaluation before concluding that the scoliosis is idiopathic.

Treatment assumes that a progressive scoliosis will cause unacceptable deformities, an increased risk of early joint disease and cardiorespiratory compromise. In idiopathic structural scoliosis, the risk of progression depends upon sex, age, pubertal status and the degree of curvature. Premenarchal girls are at highest risk. All patients with, or at risk of, structural scoliosis should be monitored regularly. Bracing and surgical correction are the two treatment options. Surgery is recommended earlier in those with neuromuscular or congenital scoliosis.

 KEY POINTS

- Scoliosis is often picked up incidentally and most are postural.
- Patients found to have a structural scoliosis must have a thorough neurological evaluation although most cases are idiopathic.
- A structural scoliosis in a premenarchal girl is the most likely to progress.

NEUROLOGY

CASE 61: A FITTING CHILD

History

Tom is a 4-year-old child known to have epilepsy. He is admitted to the resuscitation room in A&E with a fit. He was born at 26 weeks' gestation and had a periventricular haemorrhage which has led to moderate learning difficulties. He has had a runny nose, a cough and a fever in the last few days. The coughing sometimes leads to vomiting and his mother states that he has vomited up several of his drug doses in the last few days. He is on sodium valproate and lamotrigine. He has had previous admissions with fits but his mother says this is his longest fit. She has already administered buccal midazolam at home with no effect. No one in the family has had cold sores in the past few weeks.

Examination

Tom is in the midst of having a generalized fit which started 35 min before he reached hospital. His temperature is 40.2°C, oxygen saturation is 90 per cent in air, respiratory rate 30/min, heart rate 180/min, blood pressure 105/77 mmHg and peripheral capillary refill 5s.

He has a runny nose and an erythematous pharynx with enlarged but non-pustular tonsils. His chest is clear. He has no neck stiffness or rash. There are no other signs.

High-flow (15 L/min) 100 per cent facemask oxygen elevates the saturation to 97 per cent and an intravenous injection of lorazepam terminates the fit after a further 5 min, following which Tom is postictal.

INVESTIGATIONS		
		Normal
Haemoglobin	11.7 g/dL	11.5–15.5 g/dL
White cell count	24.4×10^9/L	$5.5–15.5 \times 10^9$/L
Neutrophils	19.2×10^9/L	$1.5–8.0 \times 10^9$/L
Platelets	435×10^9/L	$150–400 \times 10^9$/L
Urea and electrolytes	Normal	
Bone chemistry	Normal	
Liver function tests	Normal	
Glucose	7.1 mmol/L	3.5–6.5 mmol/L
C-reactive protein (CRP)	106 mg/L	<6 mg/L
Venous gas:		
pH	7.26	7.35–7.45
Pa_{CO_2}	6.8 kPa	4.7–6.4 kPa
Pa_{O_2}	3.1 kPa	11–14.4 kPa
HCO_3	19 mmol/L	22–29 mmol/L
Base excess	−7 mmol/L	(−3)–(+3) mmol/L

Questions
- What is the most likely cause of this child's prolonged fit?
- Would you do a lumbar puncture (LP)?
- What further treatment is required?

ANSWER 61

The most likely cause is poorly controlled epilepsy. A fever (secondary to an upper respiratory tract infection in this case) can decrease the threshold for a fit in a child with epilepsy. The vomiting of medication would further increase the risk of a fit. There would be no point doing drug levels in this case. The absence of neck stiffness and a rash would go against meningitis. Encephalitis is rare. There is no history of recent herpetic cold sores in the family. Encephalitis is often accompanied by a focal fit or focal neurological signs as well as a diminished conscious level and a fever. An LP should not be performed because of the length of the fit.

Although this child's fit is probably due to his epilepsy, the possibility of meningitis or encephalitis cannot be totally ruled out. He has a very high temperature, poor peripheral perfusion, has had his longest ever fit, has a raised white cell count with a neutrophilia and a raised CRP. An LP would help diagnose meningitis and encephalitis and would identify the organism and its sensitivities. However, it should not be performed if there is a risk of raised intracranial pressure, as it may lead to coning and death. A magnetic resonance imaging (MRI) or computed tomography (CT) scan may need to be performed to help rule out raised intracranial pressure prior to an LP. Furthermore, an LP often does not alter the initial management and can be done the next day if the patient is better, in order to elucidate the diagnosis and help determine the type and length of antimicrobial treatment.

> **!** Relative contraindications to a lumbar puncture (reproduced with modifications from APLS manual, agreed by ALSG and Blackwell Publishing 2005):
>
> - Prolonged or focal seizure
> - Focal neurological signs
> - A widespread purpuric rash
> - A Glasgow Coma Scale score <13
> - Abnormal posture or movement e.g. decerebrate posture
> - An inappropriately low pulse, raised blood pressure and irregular breathing (suggesting impending brain herniation)
> - Thrombocytopenia or clotting disorder
> - Pupillary dilatation
> - Papilloedema
> - Hypertension

Intravenous fluids, initially 0.9 per cent saline 20 ml/kg, should be administered to improve perfusion and to help normalize the capillary refill time. Intravenous ceftriaxone, clarithromycin and aciclovir should be administered. Antipyretics should also be given. Clinical progress and an LP when the patient is better will help determine the diagnosis and the necessary treatment.

Measuring the blood glucose at the bedside is essential to rule out hypoglycaemia in fitting children. One should never give more than a total of two doses of benzodiazepines, because of the risk of respiratory depression. Status epilepticus is one of the commonest paediatric emergencies and it is important to be familiar with its treatment.

 KEY POINTS

- A glucose level should always be measured in a fitting child.
- A lumbar puncture should not be performed if there is concern about raised intracranial pressure, e.g. papilloedema or coma.

CASE 62: A FEBRILE, DROWSY CHILD

History

Alison is a 9-year-old girl who is referred to the A&E department by her GP. She was seen in surgery a few days ago with a temperature and a widespread non-specific rash, and a diagnosis of a probable viral infection was made. Her temperature has persisted although the rash is fading. Today she has been complaining of worsening headache, dislike of light and pain in her neck, back and legs. Her mother has found it difficult to wake her and she has been a bit confused. She has vomited twice and, most unusually, wet the bed. She has no significant past medical history and is taking no regular medication. She is fully immunized. Her mother has recurrent cold sores, the last about 2 weeks ago. Nobody in the family is unwell or taking medications. Her school progress is good.

Examination

Alison is lying in bed in a darkened room with her eyes closed. She is reluctant to be examined and wants to go back to sleep. Her temperature is 39.7°C. She has a fading macular rash over her trunk, back, arms and legs. Her pulse is 130 beats/min. Her BP is 85/60 mmHg and the capillary refill time <2 s. There are no murmurs. She has moderate neck stiffness. She is difficult to wake but when she does she recognizes her parents but appears disorientated, thinking that she is at home. There are no focal neurological signs. Examination of the respiratory, abdominal and ENT systems is normal.

🔍 INVESTIGATIONS		
Haemoglobin	12.6 g/dL	11.5–15.5 g/dL
White cell count	11.2 × 10⁹/L	4.5 – 13.5 × 10⁹/L
Neutrophils	5.6 × 10⁹/L	3.0–5.8 × 10⁹/L
Lymphocytes	5.0 × 10⁹/L	1.5–3.0 × 10⁹/L
Platelets	365 × 10⁹ /L	150–400 × 10⁹/L
Sodium	138 mmol/L	138–146 mmol/L
Potassium	4.5 mmol/L	3.5–5.0 mmol/L
Urea	4.2 mmol/L	1.8–6.4 mmol/L
Creatinine	46 μmol/L	27–62 μmol/L
C-reactive protein	23 mg/L	< 6 mg/L

Questions
- What is the most likely diagnosis?
- What would be your immediate management of this patient?
- What further investigations would you request and when?

ANSWER 62

The most likely diagnosis is a viral meningoencephalitis. Typically there is a prodrome of a non-specific febrile illness, possibly accompanied by a rash, followed by the onset of a progressive headache and photophobia. Any virus can be responsible, but at least 80 per cent of cases are caused by enteroviruses. Of the other infectious agents mimicking viral meningoencephalitis, by far the most important are bacteria, because they require prompt treatment with antibiotics. The other major differential is a brain abscess.

Remember the maxim 'treat the treatable'. Pending culture results, the assumption has to be that a bacterial cause is possible even when, as in this case, the blood tests are not supportive. A broad-spectrum antibiotic such as cefotaxime should be started immediately following blood cultures. Most causes of viral meningoencephalitis have no specific treatment and the management is supportive. However, herpes simplex virus type 1 (HSV-1) is an important cause (note her mother's cold sores) and without treatment 70 per cent progress to coma and death. Brain involvement is focal and patients frequently present with focal seizures. All patients with meningoencephalitis should therefore be started on aciclovir. *Mycoplasma pneumoniae* can also cause meningoencephalitis and Alison should also be treated with a macrolide antibiotic such as clarithromycin.

An EEG is valuable in supporting the diagnosis. Typically it shows slow-wave activity without focal features, except in HSV-1 infection where there may be evidence of temporal lobe involvement. A magnetic resonance imaging (MRI) or computed tomography (CT) scan may show brain swelling and is mandatory if there are focal signs. It will also exclude a brain abscess. At some stage a lumbar puncture (LP) will be necessary but it is currently contraindicated because this girl is drowsy and disorientated, is likely to have raised intracranial pressure and could cone if an LP is performed. There is no urgency because she is already receiving the appropriate treatment. Cerebrospinal fluid (CSF) analysis should help differentiate between the various potential diagnoses (see Table 62.1).

Table 62.1 Cerebrospinal fluid findings in the commonest central nervous system infections

Condition	Pressure (mmH$_2$O)	White cells (mm^3)	Protein (g/L)	Glucose (mmol/L)	Comments
Normal	50–80	<5	0.2–0.4	>70 per cent blood glucose	Clear and colourless
Viral	Normal or slightly ↑	Rarely >1000. Neutrophils early but thereafter mostly lymphocytes	0.5–2.0 Grossly ↑ in HSV	Normal	Clear. Viral culture and PCR
Bacterial	Usually ↑	100–>10 000 Mostly neutrophils	1.0–5.0	↓ <50 per cent blood glucose	Turbid. Organisms seen on Gram stain. Culture and PCR

HSV, herpes simplex virus; PCR, polymerase chain reaction.

Most patients with viral meningoencephalitis make a complete recovery, except for HSV-1 where sequelae, sometimes severe, are common.

KEY POINTS

- Patients with clinical features of meningoencephalitis should be assumed to have a bacterial cause and started immediately on appropriate antibiotics as well as aciclovir.
- An LP should not be performed on a child in a coma or with raised intracranial pressure because of the risk of coning.
- Unlike most viral causes, herpes simplex type 1 meningoencephalitis is associated with significant morbidity and mortality.

CASE 63: A BIG HEAD

History

Sami, a 9-month-old boy, has been referred to the community paediatric clinic by his health visitor because his head circumference is on the 99.6th centile. He was born at 38 weeks' gestation by spontaneous vaginal delivery, following an uneventful pregnancy to a Samoan woman. His birth weight was 4.3 kg (91st centile) and his head circumference at birth was 38 cm (98th centile). This is the mother's third baby, but the other two children have a different father. Sami doesn't sleep very well, waking up to three times per night, and this was the main reason his mother went to see her health visitor. Sami is otherwise well and has not had any previous medical problems. He has been able to sit unsupported for the last 2 months, he crawls, he can use either hand to pick up raisins or grains of rice. His mother has no concerns about his vision or hearing and he passed his newborn hearing screen. He is still breast-feeding but also eats purées and finger foods. The mother, her partner and the three children live in a two-bedroom flat. The growth chart in his parent-held child health record is shown in Figure 63.1.

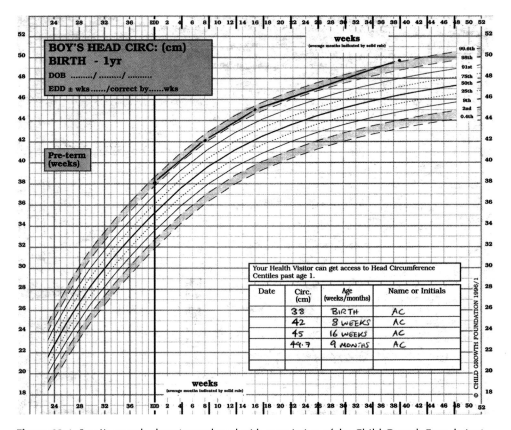

Figure 63.1 Sami's growth chart (reproduced with permission of the Child Growth Foundation).

Examination

Sami is a well-looking child, who smiles and babbles continuously. He is not dysmorphic. His weight is 10.5 kg (91st centile), his length is 76.2 cm (98th centile) and his head circumference is 49.7 cm (99.6th centile). Cardiovascular and respiratory examinations are normal. His anterior fontanelle is almost closed. Neurological examination reveals normal tone, power and reflexes in the upper and lower limbs.

Questions

- What features in the history help to distinguish between the causes of a big head?
- What other features should be sought on examination?
- What is the most likely explanation for the large head circumference?

ANSWER 63

A large head may be a normal variant, often with a familial tendency, or may be caused by pathological processes. In an infant, rising intracranial pressure will cause the skull with unfused sutures to expand rapidly. If possible, it should be determined from previous measurements whether the head circumference is enlarging and crossing centiles (a worrying feature) or whether it is just growing steadily along the same centile. There may be other symptoms of raised intracranial pressure: vomiting, lethargy, irritability, poor feeding. Developmental delay or regression (loss of previously attained developmental milestones) suggests metabolic, genetic and syndromic causes. Social concerns about a family raise the possibility of a subdural haematoma from non-accidental injury. Parents should be asked whether they or the siblings have large heads – do they have difficulty buying hats to fit them?

The causes of a large head (macrocephaly) are listed below. When performing the examination, these should be borne in mind. The shape of the head, and the size, shape and patency of the fontanelles and cranial sutures should be assessed. The presence of dysmorphic features, birthmarks or other congenital anomalies should be sought. Central and peripheral nervous systems should be examined and development assessed. Weight and height should be measured and plotted on a centile chart, as should parental head circumferences.

! Causes of macrocephaly	
	Possible examination finding
Hydrocephalus	Tense fontanelle, distended scalp veins
Vascular malformations	Cranial bruit
Tumour	Abnormal neurology
Subdural haematoma	Bruising, other injuries
Fragile X syndrome	Developmental delay, large ears
Neurofibromatosis	Café-au-lait patches, axillary freckles
Overgrowth syndrome, e.g. Soto's syndrome	Developmental delay, large hands/feet
Metabolic, e.g. mucopolysaccharidoses	Developmental delay, coarse features
Familial macrocephaly	Parent has large head circumference

Sami has normal development and his growth chart shows that he has always been a large baby with a large head. The change from the 98th centile to 99.6th centile is not concerning, considering the slow rate of change and the likelihood of small errors in measurement. The cause of his large head size is likely to be familial and this was supported by his mother's head circumference lying on the 98th centile.

KEY POINTS

- The commonest cause of a large head is familial macrocephaly.
- Check the growth chart and developmental history for a child with a big head.

CASE 64: A CHILD IN A COMA

History

Kyle is a 7-month-old boy who presents to the A&E department of a district general hospital in a coma. He has been somewhat lethargic in the last few days, has vomited several times and has gradually got worse. His parents could not rouse him and brought him straight to A&E. There is no past medical history of note and no diseases run in the family.

Examination

His airway and breathing are stable. Oxygen saturation is 96 per cent in air. His pulse is 176 beats/min, his blood pressure is 82/56 mmHg and the capillary refill is 5 s. The AVPU score is P. He is apyrexial and has no rash. The anterior fontanelle is bulging with distended veins over the scalp. There are no focal neurological signs and no other signs.

INVESTIGATIONS		
		Normal
Haemoglobin	9.6 g/dL	10.5–14.0 g/dL
White cell count	9.2×10^9/L	$4.0–11.0 \times 10^9$/L
Platelets	332×10^9/L	$150–400 \times 10^9$/L
Clotting	Normal	
Urea and electrolytes	Normal	
Liver function tests	Normal	
Bone	Normal	
Glucose	5.6 mmol/L	3.5–7 mmol/L
C-reactive protein	4 mg/L	<6 mg/L
Lactate	3.6 mmol/L	1.1–2.3 mmol/L
Ammonia	70 μmol/L	18–74 μmol/L
Capillary gas		
pH	7.35	7.36–7.44
P_{O_2}	3.1 kPa	(note capillary sample)
P_{CO_2}	6.2 kPa	4.0–6.5 kPa
Base excess	−7.2	(−2.5)–(+2.5) mmol/L
CT scan – see Figure 64.1		

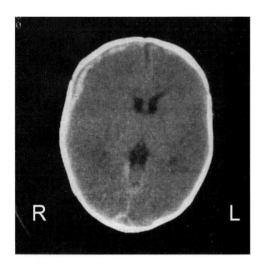

Figure 64.1 Kyle's CT scan. Reproduced with kind permission from Campbell and McIntosh (Eds). *Forfar and Arneil's Textbook of Paediatrics*. Churchill Livingstone 1998.

Questions
- What is the differential diagnosis of coma?
- What is the AVPU score?
- What does the CT scan show?
- What is the most likely mechanism?
- What is the initial medical management?

ANSWER 64

> **!** **Differential diagnosis of coma in children**
>
> - Hypoxic-ischaemic brain injury, e.g. following a respiratory arrest
> - Epileptic seizure/postictal state
> - Trauma, e.g. intracranial haemorrhage, cerebral oedema
> - Infections, e.g. meningitis, encephalitis, abscess
> - Metabolic – renal and hepatic failure, hypoglycaemia, diabetic ketoacidosis, inborn errors
> - Poisoning
> - Vascular lesions, e.g. stroke

The AVPU score is a score used for the rapid assessment of the conscious level of a child (especially <5 years of age). A = Alert, V = responds to Voice, P = responds only to Pain, U = Unresponsive to all stimuli. P or less corresponds to a GCS of 8 or less.

The CT shows an acute subdural haemorrhage over the right hemisphere.

The most likely mechanism is a shaking injury (the 'shaken baby syndrome') or possibly a direct impact.

The pulse is raised and the capillary refill time is prolonged. This would fit in with an intracranial bleed and vomiting (note the haemoglobin is low and the lactate and base excess are raised due to poor perfusion). A bolus of 20 mL/kg of 0.9 per cent saline should therefore be administered. In any child with an AVPU score of P or U, the airway is at risk and an anaesthetist should therefore be called.

A broad-spectrum antibiotic, e.g. cefotaxime, should be given as soon as possible to cover the possibility of sepsis.

The bulging anterior fontanelle indicates raised intracranial pressure. In infants, unfused sutures and a patent anterior fontanelle allow the cranial volume to increase. Raised intracranial pressure is therefore better tolerated in its initial stages and large bleeds may occur before neurological features develop. Management of raised intracranial pressure includes sitting the infant at a 30° angle, restricting fluids to two-thirds maintenance, and elective intubation and ventilation to maintain the PCO_2 at 4–4.5 kPa (intubation will also secure the airway and help ensure a safe transfer). The child should also be well oxygenated and normoglycaemic. An urgent discussion needs to be held with the regional neurosurgical centre to discuss whether the infant should be administered mannitol or hypertonic saline to help decrease the intracranial pressure. Arrangements will need to be made for an urgent neurosurgical assessment to determine whether surgery is required to evacuate the haematoma.

This injury is most likely to have been intentional. Social services should therefore be contacted and child protection procedures followed.

 KEY POINTS

- Urgent transfer of acutely ill children with an intracranial bleed to a neurosurgical unit is mandatory, as a haematoma may need to be surgically evacuated.
- The majority of serious intracranial injuries in the first year of life are the result of non-accidental injury.

History

Justin is an 18-month-old boy referred to the community paediatric clinic because he is not yet walking. He is the first child of white British parents, born at 41 weeks' gestation following an uneventful pregnancy. There was meconium staining of the amniotic fluid but he cried immediately at birth and didn't need any resuscitation. He has been generally healthy apart from normal coughs and colds, and he had chickenpox 6 months ago. His parents recall that he could roll over at about 4 months, sat up alone at 10 months, crawled from 13 months and was able to 'bear walk' on hands and feet and pull himself to standing from around 17 months. He can take a few steps holding on to furniture but cannot walk independently yet. He is able to scribble with a crayon with either hand and can slot pieces into a shape-sorter toy. He uses lots of single words appropriately, understands simple instructions, feeds himself with a spoon and will also feed his teddy bear. The parents have no concerns about his vision or hearing. He attends nursery 3 days per week and is described by the nursery staff as a likeable boy, although they have been concerned that he still doesn't walk. There is no family history of delayed walking. Justin's mother is an accountant and his father is an architect and both are in their early 40s. They are hoping to have another child soon.

Examination

Justin looks well and enjoys interacting with you. He is not dysmorphic. His weight is 10.8 kg (25th centile), height is 80 cm (25th centile) and head circumference is 49 cm (50th centile). Cardiovascular, respiratory and abdominal examinations are normal. His spine and joints appear normal, and there are no unusual birthmarks. Neurological examination shows normal cranial nerves and normal posture, tone, power and reflexes in the upper and lower limbs. He does not have any tremor. When he is helped to stand, holding on to the side of a low table, Justin takes a few steps whilst holding on with both hands.

Questions

- What comments can you make about Justin's developmental history?
- What further assessment is necessary?
- What is the most important investigation to perform?
- What are the most common causes of delayed walking?

ANSWER 65

Justin's gross motor development is delayed. Although he rolled at the normal age, he was slightly late to sit independently and crawl. The average age for walking is 13 months (range 9–18 months) and failure to walk by 18 months is a developmental warning sign. The rest of his development seems appropriate for his current age, although there is little detail given. Further assessment of his development in fine motor, speech, language, communication and social domains will reveal whether he has isolated delay in walking or he has other areas of delay too.

The most important investigation is a blood test for creatine kinase (CK) measurement. This is because boys with Duchenne muscular dystrophy (DMD) will have a very elevated CK and the diagnosis would be strongly suspected if this were found. As Justin's parents are planning to have another child, they could have appropriate genetic counselling about the risk of another child being affected. DMD is an X-linked recessive condition affecting about 1:4000 births and it usually results in progressive muscle weakness, loss of ambulation and death in the teens or early 20s. Many children with DMD will also have a degree of learning difficulty and may exhibit delay in other areas of development.

Delayed walking is a common problem. Ninety-seven per cent of normal children will be walking by 18 months of age, which means 3 per cent will not. Most children not walking by 18 months will be normal, but up to 10 per cent will have an underlying neurological problem and 10 per cent will have developmental delay in other areas. Less than 1 per cent will turn out to have muscular dystrophy.

!	**Causes of delayed walking**	
	Example
Generalized developmental delay	Fragile-X syndrome, Down's syndrome
Neuromuscular cause	Cerebral palsy, Duchenne muscular dystrophy
Musculoskeletal	Congenital dislocation of the hip
Normal 'late walker'	The majority of cases

 KEY POINTS

- Failure to walk by 18 months is a developmental warning sign.
- Duchenne muscular dystrophy is the most important diagnosis to exclude in boys.

History

Simon is 7 years old. He has been brought to the community paediatric clinic at the local children's centre by his mother and grandmother. He was referred for a medical assessment to help prepare a statement of special educational needs. His notes indicate that he has been seen previously at the children's centre by speech and language therapists due to speech delay, and by the occupational therapist because he was very clumsy. The correspondence indicates that a lot of appointments were missed and eventually he was lost to follow-up. He is the second child of non-consanguineous parents. He attends the same main-stream school as his 9-year-old brother, who has no problems at school. His father works as a delivery driver but his mother does not work. Simon was born at term and has long-standing problems with eczema and constipation. He was admitted to hospital once after scalding himself with boiling water from a kettle. He is reported to be fully immunized, although his Red Book has been lost. His mother has difficulty recalling his developmental milestones, but thinks that he walked at about 20 months and spoke his first word at about 30 months. He managed to potty-train at about 4.5 years, although he still soils himself occasionally. He used to be a contented child who would sit quietly for long periods, but his behaviour became increasingly aggressive when he started school. His mother thinks his eyesight is fine and his hearing is fine when he wants to listen. His mother and grandmother think that, overall, he is a slow learner, but they aren't particularly worried about him.

Examination

Simon appears quite slight for his age, his height is 115 cm (ninth centile) and his weight is 18 kg (second centile). He has quite a long, thin face and large ears but otherwise looks similar to his mother. He sits quietly beside his mother through most of the consultation. He speaks very little voluntarily and generally answers questions with a 'yes' or a 'no'. Cardiovascular, respiratory and abdominal examinations are normal. Neurological exam-ination reveals normal tone, power and reflexes in the upper and lower limbs. He has rather flat feet, and his knees hyperextend when standing still. His gait is normal, but he cannot stand on one leg for more than a few seconds and he seems quite clumsy when running. His eye movements and facial movements appear normal. He will not tolerate fundoscopy and is generally uncooperative with further cranial nerve assessment.

Questions
- What is a statement of educational needs?
- What further assessment is important?
- What causes should be considered for Simon's problems?

ANSWER 66

If a child's school cannot provide all of their needs, the local authority may carry out an assessment to find out what the child's special educational needs (SEN) are and how they can be supported. The findings are documented in a statement of SEN (usually just called a 'statement'). This describes the child's SEN and the assistance he or she requires. The process requires assessments by the child's school, an educational psychologist, a doctor and other relevant professionals.

The medical assessment should identify any features that may indicate specific underlying diagnoses, look for any treatable contributing factors and describe the child's current level of function and medical needs. It is essential to check hearing and vision.

The history suggests Simon may have developmental delay in multiple areas and he probably has global learning disability. He may have ligamentous laxity, with associated dyspraxia. He has chronic eczema and constipation, which may affect his ability to participate fully at school. His behavioural problems may be secondary to his learning difficulties and frustration at school, or may be an independent problem. Fragile X syndrome and Duchenne muscular dystrophy need to be considered as underlying diagnoses, but much more assessment is also needed.

❗ Examples of causes of learning difficulties

Congenital causes
- Chromosome disorder
- Fragile X syndrome
- Duchenne muscular dystrophy
- Congenital infection
- Fetal alcohol syndrome

Acquired causes
- Traumatic brain injury
- Meningitis
- Psychosocial deprivation

❗ Examples of contributing factors in learning difficulties

Problem	Solution
Hearing impairment	Hearing aids, specialist teaching
Visual impairment	Glasses, modification of classroom
Chronic medical condition	Optimize medical care
Epilepsy	Make diagnosis, anti-epileptic drugs
Autistic spectrum disorders	Specific teaching strategies
Dyspraxia	Occupational therapy
Neglect	Intervention by social services

🔑 KEY POINTS

- Children with learning difficulties may need a statement of special educational needs.
- There may be remediable problems contributing to a child's overall difficulties, e.g. deafness.

History

Leroy is a 2.5-year-old West Indian boy brought to the A&E department by ambulance. He was in the children's playground at the park apparently fit and well. He suddenly fell over whilst running to his mother and when he tried to get up, his right arm and leg were not moving and he was unable to speak. His speech has returned a little but is still far from normal and he is still not using his right side. He recognizes his parents but is a little drowsy. He is visibly upset. Nothing like this has ever happened before and his development to date has been normal. He is right-handed. Leroy was born at term following an uneventful pregnancy to healthy, unrelated parents. Apart from an orchidopexy at 13 months, he has no significant past medical history. He is on no regular medication and has no known allergies. He has two older sisters.

Examination

Leroy is a generally healthy Afro-Caribbean boy. His airway is patent and he is breathing without support. His oxygen saturation is 100 per cent in 15L of oxygen via face mask. His pulse is 92 beats/min and regular with a capillary refill time of <2s. His blood pressure is 80/54 mmHg. His temperature is 37°C. Examination of the cardiovascular, respiratory and abdominal systems is normal. He is quite sleepy but knows his parents and responds appropriately to attempts to examine him. He has drooping of the right side of his mouth but his right eye closes when he cries. He will reach out with his left hand to his favourite toy when it is held to his left but ignores it if it is introduced from his right-hand side until it is almost in the midline. Tone, power, sensation and reflexes are normal on his left side. He has increased tone in his right arm and leg but power is weak. Reflexes are brisk throughout his right side. His plantar is flexor on the left but extensor on the right.

Questions

- What is the clinical diagnosis?
- List the possible causes
- What important and relevant screening test would he have had as a neonate?
- What investigation does he need?
- What are the key points in the acute and long-term management?

ANSWER 67

Leroy has an acute right hemiplegia and hemianopia. He has an upper motor neurone VIIth nerve palsy as evidenced by eye closure despite weakness of the facial muscles. The clinical diagnosis is an acute stroke. Most childhood strokes are due to arterial occlusion (thrombotic or embolic), but venous thrombosis and haemorrhage do occur. The commonest cause of childhood stroke is sickle cell disease (SCD), affecting at least 10 per cent of such children. Many children with stroke have another medical condition.

!	Causes of acute stroke in childhood

- Haematological abnormalities – SCD, polycythaemia, leukaemia, disorders of coagulation
- Cardiac disease – congenital, especially cyanotic and acquired, e.g. endocarditis or Kawasaki disease. Usually embolic
- Infection – meningitis, local head and neck infections or bacteraemia
- Intracerebral vascular pathology – ruptured aneurysm, arteriovenous malformation
- Autoimmune disease – systemic lupus erythematosus, juvenile idiopathic arthritis, sarcoidosis
- Metabolic disease – homocystinuria, mitochondrial disorders
- Trauma

Sickle cell disease is now part of the neonatal screening programme. Previously all children from populations with a high incidence would be checked prior to any procedure that could precipitate a sickling crisis, such as surgery.

In acute stroke it is crucial to distinguish between ischaemic and other categories because this alters the investigations and management. A brain MRI should be undertaken as soon as possible, but if it is not available within 48 hours, a CT scan is an acceptable initial alternative. Scanning should be undertaken urgently if there is a depressed level of consciousness at presentation or a deterioration.

Further investigations will depend on the scan findings. For example, all children with arterial ischaemic stroke should have MRI angiography of the cervical and proximal intracranial arterial vasculature and cardiac echocardiography. They should also be investigated for an underlying prothrombotic tendency, such as protein C deficiency, as should those with venous thrombosis. A platelet count and clotting studies are needed in intracerebral haemorrhage.

The acute medical management aims to minimize future disability. He needs regular neurological observations and monitoring of his vital signs with urgent scanning and admission to the paediatric intensive care unit if there is deterioration. If an arterial ischaemic stroke is confirmed and haemorrhage and SCD are excluded, aspirin is started. Anticoagulation should be considered in specific circumstances, such as cerebral venous sinus thrombosis.

The long-term management of stroke is a prime example of the benefits of a systematic, multidisciplinary approach to assess and monitor the medical, social, emotional and educational needs of the child. All children should have an assessment within 72 hours of admission and the professionals involved should have early liaison with their counterparts in the community to ensure smooth transition of care. A key worker from one of the teams should coordinate the package of care and act as a central point of contact for the family.

 KEY POINTS

- MRI (or CT) scanning should be performed within 48 hours where there is a clinical diagnosis of childhood stroke.
- At least 10 per cent of patients with sickle cell disease will have a stroke during childhood.
- The management of childhood stroke should be multidisciplinary.

CASE 68: CHRONIC HEADACHES

History

Tom is a 10-year-old boy referred to outpatients by his GP with a 2-year history of recurrent headaches. He describes the pain as being of gradual onset, frontal, right-sided and throbbing. He has not noticed any visual symptoms. He takes paracetamol but it is of limited value. The headache is often preceded or accompanied by nausea and vomiting. His mother has noticed that he becomes very pale and quiet. He takes himself off to bed and sleeps for several hours after which he is fine. The episodes can last up to 12 hours. In between episodes Tom is fit and well. He is happy at school and doing well but missed 10 days last term due to headaches. He takes part in numerous after-school activities and loves performing arts, especially dance. He was admitted with a minor head injury at the age of 7 having fallen off his bike. There is no other significant past medical history and he takes no regular medication. His mother suffered with migraine as a teenager.

Examination

Tom is a healthy, well-grown boy. His height and weight are both on the 75th centiles. His pulse is 68 beats/min and regular and his blood pressure 96/58 mmHg. Examination of the cardiovascular, respiratory and abdominal systems is normal. His cranial nerves are intact and fundoscopy is unremarkable. His peripheral nervous system is normal.

Questions
- What is the most likely diagnosis?
- What is the differential diagnosis?
- What investigations would you request?
- Is there any treatment that would reduce the frequency of these episodes?

ANSWER 68

These are the characteristic features of common migraine – recurrent headache with symptom-free intervals, often unilateral, typically throbbing and accompanied by nausea and vomiting. Abdominal pain is often a feature. This is the commonest form of migraine in childhood and over 90 per cent have a family history. The diagnosis should be reconsidered if this is absent. Classic migraine has aura as an additional feature. Auras are usually visual and include small areas of visual loss in a visual field (scotoma) and brilliant white zigzag lines (fortification spectra).

Headaches are common in children and their frequency increases with age. In young children, certainly pre-school, an organic cause is highly likely.

! **Differential diagnosis of chronic headaches**

- Tension headaches – commonest of all, described as a 'band' or 'pressure' and bilateral. Usually otherwise asymptomatic. May last weeks and tend to worsen as day progresses. Child is otherwise healthy
- Sinusitis – percussing over affected sinuses causes pain and discomfort
- Refractive errors – ensure vision has been checked recently
- Raised intracranial pressure – a brain tumour is most parents' underlying worry. Unlike migraine and tension headaches, pain is worse when lying down. It is almost always accompanied by other abnormal symptoms, e.g. change in behaviour, or neurological signs, e.g. papilloedema
- Solvent or drug abuse
- Hypertension – blood pressure must be checked

A thorough history and examination are the mainstays in making a diagnosis in a child of this age and he probably needs no investigations. Obviously if there are focal neurological symptoms or signs (apart from visual aura), an MRI should be performed. Most children can lie still enough for this from about 7–8 years. Otherwise, sedation or a general anaesthetic is needed. The younger the child, the lower the threshold for scanning because an organic cause is more likely and they are poor at communicating the characteristics of their headache. His previous head injury is irrelevant and not an indication to scan.

Prevention of migraine should focus on lifestyle changes. Reassurance that there is no serious intracranial pathology is often enough to improve symptoms. Keeping a diary is a simple way to try to identify any trigger factors, including, rarely, a specific food. Blanket exclusion diets should be avoided. Stress, tiredness and anxiety are the commonest precipitants. Problems at school, including bullying, should be explored. Relaxation and biofeedback techniques may help. Finally, if all else fails, school attendance is affected and the migraines are unacceptably intrusive, prevention with drugs may be considered. There are very few well-designed clinical trials, but drugs such as propranolol (contraindicated in asthma), pizotifen and some of the newer anticonvulsants (gabapentin or topiramate) may be effective. All have side-effects.

 KEY POINTS

- Headaches in young children are more likely to be organic in origin and there is a lower threshold for scanning.
- Lifestyle changes, not drugs, should be the focus for the prevention of migraine.

History

Oliver is a 7-year-old boy who presents to a paediatric rapid referral clinic with 'a lop-sided face'. His mother noticed that he was drooling from the left side of his mouth for 2 days and his left eyelid has been droopy. When he smiles, his face becomes very asymmetric. He is otherwise well but the drooling has made eating and drinking difficult and a little embarrassing. His left eye also feels dry. The rest of the family are well but you notice that his mother is recovering from a cold sore. There is no history of travel or of any bites. He had an appendicectomy last year and had pyloric stenosis operated on in infancy.

Examination

The child's mouth droops on the left side. His smile, in particular, is asymmetric. It is well delineated with the normal facial creases on the right side of the face, but on the left side it is poorly formed and weak. He is also unable to shut his left eye. There are no other cranial nerve abnormalities and the neurological system is otherwise normal. Otoscopy is normal and his blood pressure is 107/67 mmHg. There are no other signs.

Questions

- What is the likely diagnosis?
- What is the treatment?
- What is the prognosis?

ANSWER 69

The most likely diagnosis is a left-sided Bell's palsy. This is a lower motor neurone palsy of the facial nerve. In lower motor neurone palsies, the whole side of the face is weak. Taste on the anterior two-thirds of the tongue on the involved side is lost in about half of cases and there may be facial numbness. In upper motor neurone facial nerve palsies, there is preserved forehead power and eye closure. The facial palsy is said to occur due to oedema of the facial nerve as it crosses the facial canal in the temporal bone. It may occur 2 weeks after a viral infection. Herpes simplex and varicella zoster are said to be causative. Epstein–Barr virus, Lyme disease and mumps have also been implicated.

In chronic cases, other causes, such as otitis media, hypertension, tumours (facial nerve or brain stem tumours), leukaemia and trauma, should also be considered.

If the facial palsy is thought to be due to an upper motor neurone facial palsy then cranial imaging with a magnetic resonance imaging (MRI) scan should be undertaken.

If the child presents within 1 week then steroid treatment with prednisolone 1 mg/kg once daily (up to 60 mg/day) for 7 days is effective. Treatment with other agents such as aciclovir is controversial. Some paediatricians would only administer it if there is a clear history of contact with herpes, as in our case, or varicella. Eye care is important. As it may not be possible for the child to close his eye, treatment with artificial tears such as hypromellose eye drops and taping of the eye at night may be necessary to prevent an exposure keratitis.

Most patients recover within a few weeks. Eighty-five per cent make a complete recovery, 10 per cent are left with mild facial weakness and 5 per cent are left with permanent significant facial weakness. Recovery may take up to 6 months.

 KEY POINTS

- A lower motor neurone facial palsy affects the forehead and eye as well as the lower part of the face.
- The commonest cause is a Bell's palsy.
- Treatment with steroids within 1 week of diagnosis is beneficial.

History

Archie is an 18-month-old boy who is referred by his GP to the paediatric day unit with a 1-week history of reduced mobility, worse in the previous 24 hours. His parents assumed he had had a minor injury at nursery because he has also been complaining that his back is sore, although there have been no witnessed events. The GP initially wondered about a reactive arthropathy affecting his hips because Archie also has a cold, but has sent him in because of the deterioration. Looking back, his parents think he has been a bit unsteady for a couple of months but this has been attributed to an ear infection. Archie walked confidently from 11 months and the rest of his development is normal. There is no significant past medical history or family history.

Examination

Archie is a generally healthy boy but is in some discomfort. Observing him in the playroom he needs propping up to sit and keeps his back very still and straight when he tries to move or reach for objects. There is very little spontaneous movement in either leg, worse with the left than the right, and he cannot weight-bear, crawl or pull himself to stand. He is reluctant to be examined but his cranial nerves and arms appear normal. Passive movement of his legs is normal, with a full range of movement in his joints. However, tone and power are reduced in both legs and reflexes are absent on the left and reduced on the right. There is no back tenderness. Examination of his cardiovascular and respiratory systems is normal. In his abdomen, there is a smooth, non-tender mass in the suprapubic region that appears to be arising out of the pelvis. It is dull to percussion.

INVESTIGATIONS		
		Normal
Haemoglobin	12.3 g/dL	11.5–15.5 g/dL
White cell count	8.4×10^9/L	$6.0 - 17.5 \times 10^9$/L
Platelets	365×10^9/L	$150–400 \times 10^9$/L
Sodium	138 mmol/L	138–146 mmol/L
Potassium	4.5 mmol/L	3.5–5.0 mmol/L
Urea	4.2 mmol/L	1.8–6.4 mmol/L
Creatinine	46 μmol/L	27–62 μmol/L
C-reactive protein	<6 mg/L	<6 mg/L

Questions
- What is the differential diagnosis of back pain in children?
- Which of these is most likely in this case?
- What should happen next?

ANSWER 70

Unlike adults, in whom back pain is frequently mechanical or psychological in origin, back pain in children, especially pre-adolescent, is almost always pathological. It can be difficult for children to localize pain and careful observation is crucial – children with back pain tend to maintain a straight, stiff back and refuse to bend forward to pick up objects from the floor.

! **Differential diagnosis of back pain in children**

- Developmental abnormalities – spondylolysis (defect in pars interarticularis), spondylolisthesis (spondylolysis with anterior slippage of affected vertebra), scoliosis
- Traumatic – vertebral stress fractures, muscle spasm due to overuse, e.g. in athletes and gymnasts, prolapsed intervertebral disc
- Neoplastic – primary benign or malignant vertebral or spinal cord tumours, leukaemias or lymphomas, metastases, e.g. neuroblastoma
- Infection – discitis (common before 6 years), vertebral osteomyelitis
- Rheumatological – pauciarticular juvenile rheumatoid arthritis, ankylosing spondylitis, psoriatic arthritis

---

Of these, only a prolapsed disc and tumours are associated with neurological abnormalities and the former is very rare, especially in young children. Hence a neoplastic cause is much the most likely. Archie has a flaccid paralysis of both legs with reduced or absent reflexes. The abdominal mass is probably his bladder which is neuropathic. No mention is made of any history of sphincter problems, but as he will still be in nappies this is difficult to assess. Parents may notice a reduction in the urinary stream in boys. His anus should be inspected and may be patulous. The parents should be asked about the presence of constipation. Detecting a sensory level at this age is extremely difficult.

The pointers to serious pathology in children with back pain include:

- persistent or worsening pain
- systemic features such as fever, malaise or weight loss
- neurological symptoms or signs
- sphincter dysfunction
- young age – especially <4 years when a tumour is most likely.

This is a medical emergency. If Archie is not to have permanent loss of sphincter control and irreversible damage to his legs, he needs urgent investigation and intervention to reduce cord compression. MRI is the investigation of choice and no time should be lost – hours can make a difference (see Fig. 70.1). He should be referred immediately to a paediatric neurosurgery centre. Spinal cord tumours are classified according to their anatomical location: intramedullary (within the cord), extramedullary intradural (usually benign) and extramedullary extradural (usually metastases). Further treatment and prognosis will depend upon the findings.

This boy was found to have a diffuse intramedullary spinal tumour from T7 to T12.

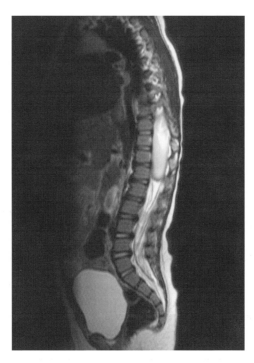

Figure 70.1 Sagittal MRI scan of Archie's spine.

He underwent limited debulking. Histology showed a low-grade pilocytic astrocytoma. Although these are slow-growing indolent tumours, it is their critical location that governs morbidity and mortality. The surgical options are limited and radiotherapy likewise. Trials of chemotherapy are in progress.

 KEY POINTS

- Back pain in children should be assumed to be organic until proven otherwise.
- To minimize irreversible damage, back pain in association with neurological abnormalities is an indication for urgent MRI scanning and referral to neurosurgery.
- Location is a key predictor of outcome in brain and spinal cord tumours.

CASE 71: DEVELOPMENTAL REGRESSION

History

Theo is a 7-month-old boy who is seen as an urgent referral in the paediatric clinic. His parents have been concerned that he has stopped interacting with them as he used to, and that he has started to have unusual repetitive movements. He was born at term by elective Caesarean section, and he had no problems in the neonatal period. His parents are not consanguineous. He smiled at 5 weeks of age and by about 4 months he could support his head well when held in a sitting position, was making lots of sounds, was interested in everything around him and was reaching to touch objects. Over the last month, he has almost stopped vocalizing, seems much less interested in his surroundings and no longer seems to be as able to support his head. About 3 weeks ago he started having clusters of jerking movements, which his parents initially thought were 'startle responses'. The movements are symmetrical and cause his arms to move in front of his body and his neck to flex.

Examination

Theo is well grown for his age, with a weight of 9 kg (75th centile), length 72 cm (75th centile) and head circumference 45 cm (50th centile). Cardiovascular, respiratory and abdominal examinations are unremarkable. Cranial and peripheral nervous system examination is normal. There are five patches of pale pigmentation on the skin of his abdomen. He is able to fix on a light source and will follow it briefly but he shows little interest in faces or interacting with toys. When placed in a sitting position, his head drops forward after a few seconds, and when placed prone he does not lift his head from the ground. He does not smile or vocalize during the consultation.

Questions

- What are the most worrying features of this history and what diagnosis do you suspect?
- What investigations should be performed in the first instance?
- What underlying diagnosis may be present?

ANSWER 71

It is clear from the history that there has been developmental regression – loss of previously attained developmental milestones. The abnormal movements are suggestive of infantile spasms, a seizure type causing contraction of axial muscles, resulting in a spectrum of abnormal movements from a small nod of the head to a full 'jack-knife spasm'. This combination makes it likely that this child has West syndrome, an epilepsy syndrome characterized by infantile spasms, developmental regression and hypsarrhythmia (a chaotic pattern) on EEG. West syndrome starts in the first year of life and can have a variety of underlying causes, including structural brain abnormalities, neurometabolic disease, neurocutaneous syndromes and acquired brain injury. The seizures are difficult to control with medication, and the developmental outlook is poor. This is not necessarily the case with all causes of developmental regression, and it is very important to try to identify any treatable underlying disease, as this may dramatically change the neurodevelopmental outlook.

! Causes of developmental regression	
	Examples
Acquired brain injury	Hypoxia, meningitis
Seizure disorders	West syndrome, Landau–Kleffner syndrome
Neurometabolic/neurodegenerative	Mitochondrial disorders, Tay–Sachs disease
Toxic substances	Heavy metal poisoning, e.g. lead
Infectious	Subacute sclerosing panencephalitis, prion disease
Pervasive developmental disorder	Autism, childhood disintegrative disorder, Rett's syndrome

In the first instance, this child will require an EEG to look for hypsarrhythmia and an MRI scan to look for structural brain abnormalities. Blood tests should include a full blood count, renal and liver function tests, calcium, phosphate, glucose, lactate, ammonia and amino acids. Urine should be sent for urine amino and organic acids. Examination with a Wood's (ultraviolet) light will help to determine if there are hypopigmented areas of skin, which may be difficult to see in normal light and could indicate an underlying neurocutaneous syndrome. Further investigations should be directed by a paediatrician with experience in neurology and epilepsy.

The presence of depigmented patches on the skin (possibly ash leaf macules) raises the possibility of tuberous sclerosis. Seizures are a common presenting feature and indicate the presence of hamartomas in the central nervous system. This neurocutaneous syndrome is autosomal dominantly inherited, although many cases are new mutations. Clinical features are due to hamartomas which occur in multiple organs, including brain, skin, eyes, kidneys and heart. Tuberous sclerosis arises from defects in either of the two genes encoding the interacting proteins (tuberin on chromosome 16, and hamartin on chromosome 9) involved in the regulation of cellular growth and differentiation. The other two most common neurocutaneous syndromes are neurofibromatosis and Sturge–Weber syndrome.

KEY POINTS

- Developmental regression requires prompt and thorough evaluation by a specialist.
- Infantile spasms are usually associated with diseases with a poor prognosis.
- Tuberous sclerosis is one of the commonest causes of developmental regression and infantile spasms.

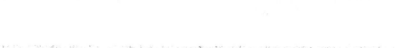

History

Ronan is a 3-year-old boy with Down's syndrome. He is brought to his GP because his parents are worried about his hearing. He does not seem to notice when his parents call his name if he is not looking directly at them, his speech has become less clear and his nursery teachers are concerned that his behaviour has become more difficult to manage. He has also started to snore when asleep.

Ronan was born at 36 weeks' gestation. He required admission to the neonatal unit for poor feeding and also needed a partial volume dilutional exchange transfusion for poly-cythaemia with hypoglycaemia and seizures. He had a normal newborn hearing screen. He has a small ventricular septal defect and he had bacterial endocarditis 6 months ago, necessitating a long course of intravenous antibiotics. His mother is a 30-year-old teacher and his father is a 43-year-old manager of a computer company. They are both well. Ronan has been fully immunized, including an influenza vaccine last winter.

Examination

Ronan's weight and length are on the 25th centile on the Down's syndrome growth chart. He smiles at you when you approach and seems to follow visual cues and be affectionate with his parents. His speech is difficult to understand. Cardiovascular exam-ination reveals a heart rate of 110 beats/min, a grade 3 pansystolic murmur, loudest at the lower left sternal edge, and no signs of cardiac failure. His respiratory and abdom-inal examinations are unremarkable. Both tympanic membranes have a dull retracted appearance with loss of the light reflex and some bubbles visible behind the membrane. He has large tonsils that almost touch in the middle.

Questions
- What is the most likely cause of his hearing difficulties?
- What other possibilities are there?
- How could his hearing be assessed?

ANSWER 72

Ronan is most likely to have conductive hearing loss secondary to chronic otitis media with an effusion (OME, or 'glue ear'). This diagnosis is consistent with the fact that his hearing has recently deteriorated, that he snores (indicating partial upper airway obstruction in sleep) and the findings on examination of his ears. Children with Down's syndrome are particularly vulnerable to OME because their large adenoids, small nasopharynx and narrow Eustachian tubes make aeration of the middle ear less efficient. For these reasons, children with Down's syndrome should have regular screening for hearing impairment.

In addition to conductive deafness, sensorineural deafness is more common in children with Down's syndrome. The normal newborn hearing screen (otoacoustic emissions) makes congenital sensorineural deafness unlikely. Sensorineural hearing loss can be acquired, and a potential risk factor is the use of aminoglycoside antibiotics, e.g. gentamicin, which may have been used in the treatment of his bacterial endocarditis. Aminoglycosides cause dose-related ototoxicity and some individuals also have an underlying genetic susceptibility. Another possibility is that Ronan has autism. This is more common in children with Down's syndrome and can present with abnormal speech, language and behaviour, which may initially be attributed to hearing difficulties.

Features of conductive and sensorineural hearing loss		
	Conductive	*Sensorineural*
Causes	Glue ear	Genetic
	Congenital ear abnormalities	Infections: congenital / postnatal
		Birth asphyxia
		Head injury
Severity	Milder; intermittent	More severe; static or progressive
	20–60 dB loss	20–120 dB loss
Management	Conservative	Hearing aid
	Grommets	Cochlear implant

Ronan should be referred urgently to a paediatric audiology clinic, so that there is minimal delay in detection of any significant hearing impairment, and to minimize further delay of his speech and language development. Ideally, he would already have regular follow-up in such a clinic. His hearing will be assessed using techniques appropriate to his developmental age. These may include visual reinforcement audiometry (where a visual signal reinforces a correct head-turning response to localize a sound), free field conditioning (where an auditory stimulus is the cue for an action in a simple game), and speech discrimination tests (where toys are named at a set volume and identified by the child). He would also have tympanometry performed to confirm negative middle ear pressures typical of OME. It would also be important to ask if Ronan has sleep apnoea, which is associated with severe upper airway obstruction and which may necessitate an adenotonsillectomy.

KEY POINTS

- It is important to recognize and refer hearing problems at an early stage.
- Conductive hearing loss due to glue ear is the most common cause of hearing impairment.
- Children with Down's syndrome have an increased risk of hearing problems and require surveillance.

CASE 73: A CHILD WITH A SQUINT

History

Rachel is a 9-month-old girl who is brought to her GP practice by her mother. Over the last month her parents have noticed that her eyes don't always seem to be looking in the same direction. She was born at 35 weeks' gestation after an emergency Caesarean section for suspected placental abruption, but was in good condition at birth. There were no medical problems after delivery. She had chickenpox 1 month ago, but has never really been to the surgery otherwise, except for her immunizations. Her mother reports that she his happy with her development, as Rachel is doing everything at about the same age that her 3-year-old brother did.

Examination

Rachel is a healthy-looking child. She has an obvious right convergent squint. Figure 73.1 illustrates the appearance of her eyes as she looks around.

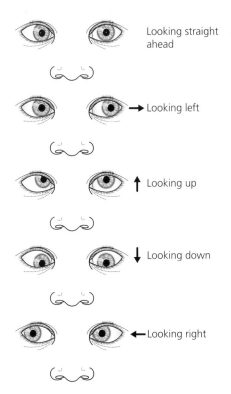

Looking straight ahead

Looking left

Looking up

Looking down

Looking right

Figure 73.1 Appearance of Rachel's eyes as she looks around.

Questions

- What is a convergent squint?
- What are the possible causes of a squint in a child this age?
- What simple assessment can be performed?
- What should be done next?

ANSWER 73

Squint (strabismus) is a common problem, which may be intermittent or constant. The visual axes of the eyes cannot be aligned simultaneously, resulting in the appearance of one eye not looking in the same direction as the other. A right convergent squint (esotropia) means that the right eye is turned in towards the nose when the left eye is looking directly at a target.

Squints may be paralytic or concomitant. Paralytic squints are caused by dysfunction of the motor nerves controlling eye movements (cranial nerves III, IV and VI). Whilst paralytic squints are rare, it is essential to recognize them, as they may be the first sign of a brain tumour or a neurological disorder. Concomitant squints are common and are usually due to extraocular muscle imbalance in infants, or refractive errors after infancy. The most common manifestation is the squinting eye turning medially. A concomitant squint can also be the presenting feature of more serious eye disease, such as retinoblastoma. Rachel has a concomitant squint.

A squint can be confirmed by testing the corneal light reflex – shining a point light source to produce a reflection on both corneas and looking at the position of the reflection on each eye. Sometimes prominent epicanthic folds or a broad nasal bridge will create the impression of a squint (pseudosquint), but in this case the light reflex will be normal. The range of eye movements should be tested by moving a visual stimulus to determine if there is a paralytic squint – the affected eye will not be able to follow the stimulus in all directions. The red reflexes should be tested with an ophthalmoscope. Absence of the red reflex indicates ocular pathology such as a cataract or retinoblastoma.

The cover test (see Fig. 73.2) should be performed to determine the nature of the squint. Whilst the child looks at a visual stimulus, each eye is covered in turn. The observer looks at the movement of the uncovered eye first, and then the covered eye as it is uncovered. When the fixing eye is covered, the squinting eye will move to take over fixation. Sometimes a squint may only be apparent when an eye is covered (latent squint) and this can be inferred from movement of the eye as it is uncovered.

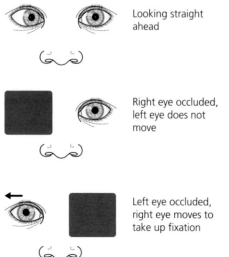

Looking straight ahead

Right eye occluded, left eye does not move

Left eye occluded, right eye moves to take up fixation

Figure 73.2 Cover test.

Mild and intermittent squint may be present in the neonatal period and disappear without treatment. Any child over 3 months of age with a squint, or parental concern about a squint, should be referred to an orthoptist or ophthalmologist for further assessment. The aim is to detect any serious underlying pathology and to prevent the development of amblyopia. In the developing brain, the image from the squinting eye is suppressed to avoid diplopia. In an untreated squint, this leads to irreversible suppression of the visual pathways, visual impairment in that eye and possible blindness. This phenomenon is known as amblyopia. Treatments include correction of refractive errors with glasses, patching of the good eye to force use of the other eye, and surgery on the extraocular muscles.

 KEY POINTS

- Squint is a common childhood problem.
- It is essential to determine if it is a paralytic or non-paralytic squint.
- Referral to a specialist is important to prevent development of amblyopia.

CHILD AND ADOLESCENT PSYCHIATRY

CASE 74: A BOY WITH NO FRIENDS

History

Adrian is a 10-year-old boy with difficult behaviour at home, who comes for a review to the community paediatric clinic. He was thought to have attention deficit hyperactivity disorder (ADHD) after an initial consultation in the clinic. However, information obtained from his school indicated that his teacher did not find his behaviour to be hyperactive or inattentive. His mother had mentioned that he didn't seem to have any friends to play with and that this seemed to be the reason he was always causing trouble at home. It is decided that it might be helpful to observe his behaviour in school.

You observe Adrian at school over a 2-hour period. He does not know that you are specifically watching him. Initially he has a games lesson: the children are practising football skills. Adrian seems interested, but whenever the task involves a complex instruction, he doesn't seems to be able to follow it. When this happens, he stands still or does his own thing. He doesn't ask anyone else to explain what he is supposed to do. He doesn't join in with the playground banter between the other children and the teacher. At the end of the lesson, there is a short game of football and he is the last to be picked for a team. He seems to find it hard to anticipate the flow of the game and runs around almost aimlessly. When he does get the ball he runs straight down the pitch with it and ends up colliding with another child who is trying to tackle him.

Next he is observed in the classroom, where he is doing mathematics. Again he participates very little in the classroom discussion and he doesn't really speak to the other children. He sits quietly, fidgets and slouches frequently, but doesn't leave his seat. He places his pens and ruler in a neat row and gets quite upset when another child borrows his ruler and disrupts the pattern. When he is asked a question, he mumbles only half of the answer. His book shows that he has worked out most of the simple sums correctly but has struggled with the questions that required more reasoning.

His teacher reports that the staff find Adrian quite bewildering. Frequently he just doesn't understand the task he is asked to do and he often does his own thing, but sometimes he is able produce complex pieces of work. Even with one-to-one teaching it has been impossible to determine his true academic potential, and sometimes he gets very upset when teachers try to give him extra guidance. His social interaction is always odd, he doesn't have any real friends, and although the other children will tolerate him joining in their games, this frequently results in trouble. Sometimes he will just play on his own, e.g. opening and closing the lock on the playground gate. He won't participate in discussions or drama and when he does speak in front of the class he may speak with a strange intonation or say things that are not appropriate to the context. He gets very anxious about apparently minor things such as changes in the day's timetable. Last week he got upset several times each day because the classroom clock had not been set to the right time.

Questions

- What underlying causes may explain Adrian's problems?
- What additional assessment would be helpful?
- How might making a diagnosis help Adrian to achieve his full potential at school?

ANSWER 74

Adrian displays evidence of difficulties with social communication, social interaction and obsessional behaviour. He may have an autistic spectrum disorder, possibly Asperger's syndrome. This diagnosis cannot be made with certainty from the brief history, and further assessment would be needed. Other underlying or contributing problems might include hearing difficulties, specific learning difficulties, social and emotional problems.

Autism is characterized by the triad of impairment of social communication, social interaction and rigidity of thought and behaviour. Unusual routines and interests, abnormal sensory sensitivity and learning or other developmental difficulties may coexist. The term autistic spectrum disorder is now widely accepted and recognizes that there can be considerable variation in the severity of symptoms.

Autistic disorder is the most severe end of the spectrum and is usually diagnosed in early childhood. Affected children are often non-verbal, with cognitive impairment and highly stereotyped behaviours. At the milder end of the spectrum there may be relatively little impairment of communication, leading to a diagnosis being made later in life, if at all. Asperger's syndrome is at the mild end of the autistic spectrum and individuals are usually of average or above-average intelligence, have difficulties understanding non-verbal communication cues, find it difficult to form friendships and difficult to empathize with others. Autistic spectrum disorders may affect up to 1 per cent of children in the UK.

Additional assessment should include a hearing test and assessment by a paediatrician with an interest in autistic spectrum disorders (usually a community paediatrician) or a child and adolescent mental health team. Often a clinical psychologist or a multidisciplinary team of other professionals will be involved in the assessment. Detailed developmental, medical, family and social histories should be taken. Adrian's social skills, communication and behaviour will be observed. Sometimes this is done in a standardized way using an observational assessment. The process needs the support of the family, who should understand that the eventual outcome might be a diagnosis of autistic spectrum disorder.

Making a diagnosis of autistic spectrum disorder can be very emotive. It can bring great relief to parents and the child, but can also be met with denial or dismay. Understanding the diagnosis will enable the teachers at Adrian's school to understand why he behaves in the way he does. It will allow the school to implement strategies to help Adrian to be included as fully as possible in the curriculum. This will include individualized measures to support social communication and behavioural interventions to assist the development of adaptive skills. The special educational needs coordinator at the school will help to develop an individual education plan to help staff to know what Adrian's needs are and how they can best be met.

 KEY POINTS

- Autism is characterized by impairments of social communication, social interaction and rigidity of thought and behaviour.
- Autistic spectrum disorders may remain undiagnosed in late childhood and adolescence.
- Making the diagnosis may help to find strategies to improve learning and behaviour.

History

Richard is a 6-year-old boy who is brought to the community paediatric clinic by his mother. She asked her GP to refer Richard because she thinks he is hyperactive. She describes him as 'always on the go', unable to sit still or concentrate on anything, and never seeming to think before he acts. He is particularly difficult at home in the evenings and rarely goes to bed before midnight. His behaviour has been getting worse over the last year. His mother says that she just can't cope with his behaviour any more and would like him to be put on some medicine to calm him down.

Richard was born at 35 weeks' gestation, and his only medical problem has been eczema. This has been difficult to control and he is under follow-up by a paediatric dermatologist. He currently uses a combination of emollients and a topical steroid. He has two teenage half-brothers and a 1-year-old half-sister. His mother is separated from her partner and now looks after the children alone. She works part-time as a beautician. The family lives in a small flat and Richard attends his local primary school. There have been problems with anti-social neighbours, and Richard's oldest brother has recently been in trouble with the police.

Richard sits quietly whilst his mother gives this history. When asked directly, he says that he enjoys school and gets on well with his brothers and sister. He misses his father, whom he doesn't see anymore. His mother says that he's better behaved when he is outside the home, and other people don't see what he's really like.

Questions
- What is attention deficit hyperactivity disorder (ADHD)?
- What additional questions will help to determine if this is the diagnosis?
- What treatment can be used for ADHD?

ANSWER 75

Attention deficit hyperactivity disorder is characterized by inattention, hyperactivity and/or impulsiveness, which are excessive for the child's developmental age and cause significant social or academic problems. The problems must have begun before 7 years of age, have been present for at least 6 months, and must be present in more than one setting, which usually means at home and at school. Children often appear to be constantly 'on the go', fidgety, unable to sustain concentration or organize themselves and unable to wait their turn. ADHD affects 2–5 per cent of school-age children with boys four times more commonly affected. In later life it is associated with an increased risk of unemployment, criminality and substance misuse.

Many children have behaviour which overlaps with some of the features of ADHD. It is important to distinguish between overactivity, one end of the normal spectrum, and hyperactivity. Rarely, a physical disorder such as thyrotoxicosis will be misdiagnosed as ADHD. In Richard's case the history indicates that there are lots of potential psycho-social and emotional stresses that could cause difficult behaviour: a new sister, separated parents, a mother trying to divide her attention between four children of very different ages, disturbances by neighbours, poor sleep and a chronic medical problem.

It is important to establish when the problems first started, and how the behaviour problems have evolved in each of the domains of inattention, hyperactivity and impulsiveness. It is essential to discover whether the problems also occur at school, and this is best done by contacting Richard's teacher (with parental consent). There are standardized questionnaires that can be completed by parents and teachers to assess his behaviour more objectively. More family and social history will be useful to determine the impact of all of the different stresses in his life. His bedtime routine and sleep patterns need to be addressed because children who do not get enough sleep can often behave in a hyperactive way. Richard's progress at school, his development and his hearing need to be carefully assessed. Finally, his mother's agenda must be explored. Often the child's behaviour is more of a problem for the parents than the child. In fact, Richard's behaviour at school was fairly normal and he did not have ADHD. His problems were attributed to his family circumstances and dynamics, and he was referred to a child psychologist.

Treatments for ADHD are pharmacological and behavioural. Paradoxically, stimulant medication helps to keep the child focused on a task and relieves many of the symptoms of ADHD. Methylphenidate is the usual first choice, but should only be commenced under specialist supervision. Side-effects include loss of appetite, poor sleep and abdominal pain. Behavioural treatment aims to help the child and family modify their behaviour to minimize the impact of ADHD. Changes to how the child is dealt with in the home and school environments may be needed.

 KEY POINTS

- Attention deficit hyperactivity disorder (ADHD) is a common condition.
- Similar symptoms can have many other causes.
- Stimulant medication should only be commenced under specialist supervision.

CASE 76: A TEENAGER WHO WON'T EAT

History

Claire is a 15-year old girl who is urgently referred to the paediatric clinic because of weight loss, nausea and a poor appetite. She is accompanied by her mother and father, who do most of the talking. They were shocked when they took her on holiday 3 weeks ago and they saw how little Claire ate. When they forced her to join them for meals in restaurants, she complained of feeling sick and having no appetite. She has become an increasingly picky eater over the last year or so, first becoming vegetarian and then rarely eating with her parents because mealtimes clashed with her running training. During that time she became the county cross-country running champion, and she trains at least once every day. Her mother thinks she goes to the toilet more often than normal and is worried that she has not menstruated for the last 4 months. Claire has lost a lot of weight and all her clothes from 1 year ago are very loose on her.

Claire is quiet while her parents talk, but when asked directly she says that she doesn't think there is a problem. She says that she has lost some weight over the last year, but that was necessary for her running. She eats when she is hungry and is very careful about her diet because she needs the right foods to optimize her performance. She says that she feels healthier than she ever has, although she admits that her running performance has deteriorated over the last two months. She enjoys her school, works hard and achieves top grades. She says that things are fine at home and that her parents should be proud of her rather than worried. She is quite pleased that she hasn't menstruated for 4 months as periods are quite a nuisance. She says she is not sexually active and denies any drug use. She is otherwise healthy and just takes laxatives occasionally for constipation. She has a 12-year-old brother whom she likes. Her father manages his own company and her mother is a dance teacher.

Examination

Claire's weight is 39 kg (< second centile) and her height is 166 cm (75th centile). Her skin is dry and her bones appear very prominent. She has fine downy hair over her face. Her heart rate is 55 beats/min and regular, but otherwise cardiovascular, respiratory, abdominal and ear, nose and throat examinations are normal.

Questions
- What is Claire's body mass index?
- What is the most likely diagnosis and what questions would help to confirm this?
- What other diagnoses must be considered?
- What physical complications can arise from this condition?

ANSWER 76

Body mass index (BMI) is calculated as weight (kg)/height^2 (m^2). Claire's BMI is 14.2 kg/m^2. BMI centile charts are available for boys and girls and demonstrate the variation with age. A BMI less than the fifth centile is considered underweight, and Claire falls well below this.

The most likely diagnosis is anorexia nervosa. Claire is severely underweight, she exercises excessively, may abuse laxatives, has secondary amenorrhoea and denies the seriousness of the problem. Specific questions about her attitude to her body shape, eating and weight gain should be asked. Symptoms of depression and obsessive compulsive disorder should be sought, as these may coexist with anorexia.

Other diagnoses to consider include thyrotoxicosis, inflammatory bowel disease and bulimia nervosa, although none of these would have all of the features described above.

! Features of anorexia nervosa and bulimia nervosa

Anorexia nervosa	*Bulimia nervosa*
Body weight well below normal	Body weight normal or overweight
Intense fear of weight gain	Recurrent binge eating
Abnormal perception of body	Abnormal compensatory behaviour
Amenorrhoea	Fear of weight gain
Either restriction of intake or binge eating and purging	

! Physical complications of anorexia nervosa

- Cardiovascular – bradycardia, hypotension, conduction abnormalities
- Neurological – cognitive impairment, poor concentration
- Renal – fluid and electrolyte abnormalities, pre-renal failure
- Endocrine – amenorrhoea, delayed/arrested puberty, osteoporosis
- Gastrointestinal – abnormal motility and absorption, damage from purgatives
- Haematological – anaemia, thrombocytopenia, leucopenia
- Skin – dry skin, lanugo hair, brittle nails

Management of anorexia nervosa requires specialist expertise and may involve in-patient treatment to establish weight gain and to correct any dangerous metabolic derangements. During re-feeding, life-threatening changes in electrolytes and a cardio-myopathy may develop. Outpatient management tries to address the longer-term issues of abnormal body perception and fear of weight gain.

 KEY POINTS

- Anorexia nervosa is characterized by being severely underweight, a fear of weight gain and an abnormal body perception.
- Anorexia nervosa can lead to dangerous physical complications.

NEONATOLOGY

CASE 77: BORN TOO EARLY

History

Mrs Richardson is a 23-year old lady in her first pregnancy, who is admitted to hospital at 26 weeks' gestation because she has had spontaneous rupture of membranes. Forty-eight hours later she goes into spontaneous labour and a baby boy is delivered, weighing 800 g (25th centile). At delivery he is making spontaneous respiratory effort with marked subcostal and sternal recession. He is stabilized and transported to the neonatal unit.

| **INVESTIGATIONS**
|---|
| Baby Richardson's chest radiograph is shown in Figure 77.1. |

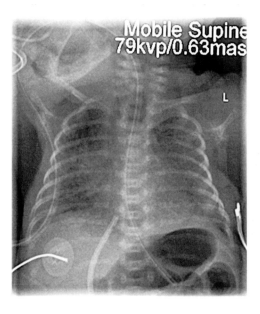

Figure 77.1 Chest radiograph at 4 hours of age.

Questions

- What can be done before delivery to optimize the outcome for a premature baby?
- What are the management priorities for the baby at delivery?
- What is the lung pathology seen in the chest radiograph?
- What complications of prematurity does this baby face?

ANSWER 77

The outcome for a baby destined to be born prematurely can be improved by the administration of corticosteroids to the mother, preferably at least 48 hours before delivery. This increases surfactant production by the fetus, reduces the risk and the severity of the respiratory distress syndrome, increases survival and reduces other morbidities. When there has been prolonged rupture of membranes, administration of antibiotics to the mother reduces the risk of sepsis in the newborn. Where possible, delivery should be planned so that the neonatal team and their equipment are fully prepared and experienced members of staff are available. The parents should be counselled about what to expect and the outcomes for a baby born prematurely. The importance of expressing breast milk as soon as possible after delivery should be emphasized.

At delivery, the immediate management priorities for a premature baby are similar to those for any other baby. However, heat loss will be greater, as they are smaller, the lungs are stiffer due to surfactant deficiency and are more fragile, and the premature baby will have fewer metabolic reserves. The baby should be dried and covered, or placed in a plastic bag under a radiant heater. The baby should be assessed for breathing, heart rate, colour and tone, and the airway positioned optimally. The baby will need respiratory support, which may be non-invasive continuous positive airways pressure (CPAP), or intubation. Surfactant may need to be administered in the delivery room. Excessive positive pressure ventilation (which may cause a pneumothorax) and hyperoxia should be avoided. The baby should then be transferred promptly to the neonatal unit.

The chest radiograph shows airspace shadowing consistent with respiratory distress syndrome (RDS, also known as hyaline membrane disease or surfactant deficiency disease). Surfactant is produced by type II pneumocytes and its production by the fetus increases towards term. Deficiency of surfactant results in poorly compliant, low-volume lungs, with ventilation–perfusion mismatching. Although surfactant production will increase after delivery, this can be impaired by acidosis, hypoxia and hypothermia. Clinical features include grunting, tachypnoea, chest recession and cyanosis. Exogenous surfactant can be administered via an endotracheal tube and can be given electively to very premature babies, who are very likely to develop RDS, or as rescue treatment when RDS becomes apparent.

! **Complications of premature birth**

- Respiratory – RDS, pneumothorax, apnoea, chronic lung disease
- Cardiovascular – patent ductus arteriosus
- Neurological – periventricular haemorrhage, periventricular leucomalacia
- Gastrointestinal – necrotizing enterocolitis, gastro-oesophageal reflux
- Infection – group B *Streptococcus*, nosocomial infection
- Metabolic – hypoglycaemia, jaundice, rickets
- Iatrogenic – extravasation injury, pressure sores

KEY POINTS

- Antenatal corticosteroids improve the outcome of premature infants.
- Respiratory distress syndrome is common in premature babies.
- Endotracheal administration of surfactant is used to treat respiratory distress syndrome.

History

You are called to the labour ward to see a full-term newborn baby boy because he has difficulty breathing. He was born 15 min ago to a 20-year-old first-time mother, who apparently had little antenatal care. The baby was born by Caesarean section because it was found to be in the breech position. The midwife said that the baby made a few cries immediately after birth, had good tone and a heart rate over 100 beats/min. She had placed him on the resuscitaire and then had to attend to the mother. When she next looked at the baby, he was breathing very fast and was making a grunting noise. The mother has mild learning difficulties but no history of any other significant medical problems or of drug use.

Examination

The baby looks an appropriate size for his gestational age, he is not dysmorphic, and he has been wrapped in a dry towel. His lips and tongue appear slightly blue. He is making an intermittent grunting expiratory sound, and his respiratory rate is 70/min. Air entry is reduced on the left side of his chest, with no increase in resonance on percussion. His heart rate is approximately 150 beats/min, his heart sounds are normal and his femoral pulses are palpable. His abdomen appears slightly concave.

He is transferred urgently to the neonatal unit and a chest radiograph (Fig. 78.1) is taken shortly afterwards.

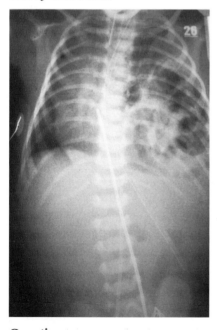

Figure 78.1 Chest radiograph of breathless newborn.

Questions

- What is the diagnosis?
- How should this newborn be managed?
- What other conditions can cause respiratory distress in a term newborn after an unremarkable delivery?

ANSWER 78

The most common cause of respiratory distress in a term baby following a Caesarean section is transient tachypnoea of the newborn due to delayed clearance of lung fluid. However, this does not produce the clinical or radiographic features seen in this case. Here the diagnosis is congenital diaphragmatic hernia. Although many cases are picked up through antenatal screening, herniation of bowel through defects in the diaphragm can occur late in gestation or even after delivery. It usually presents with respiratory distress at, or shortly after, birth. The abdomen appears concave because some of its contents are within the thorax, the mediastinum and apex beat may be displaced and bowel sounds may be heard in the chest. The chest radiograph shows mediastinal shift with air-filled bowel loops occupying the left hemithorax. The baby has been intubated, a nasogastric tube is in place, and umbilical venous and arterial catheters have been inserted.

It is important to intubate the baby early to prevent the swallowing of air, which can cause expansion of the bowel within the chest and further respiratory compromise. If the diagnosis is known before delivery, the use of bag-and-mask ventilation should be avoided for the same reason. A nasogastric tube should be placed to aspirate gastric fluid and air. Meticulous intensive care is needed to optimize the baby before surgery is performed because the lungs are usually hypoplastic (partly due to compression by bowel within the thorax) and pulmonary hypertension is a frequent complication. Mortality rates of 20 per cent are expected even with optimal care.

!   **Causes of unexpected respiratory distress in the term newborn**

- Transient tachypnoea of the newborn
- Pneumothorax
- Congenital pneumonia, sepsis
- Lung malformations, congenital diaphragmatic hernia
- Oesophageal atresia, tracheo-oesophageal fistula
- Choanal atresia, other upper airway malformations
- Congenital heart disease
- Anaemia, polycythaemia
- Cerebral haemorrhage

 KEY POINTS

- Transient tachypnoea of the newborn is the most common cause of respiratory distress in a term baby, most often following Caesarean section.
- A newborn with congenital diaphragmatic hernia should be intubated promptly to prevent swallowed air distending the bowel within the thorax.
- Prognosis in congenital diaphragmatic hernia is mainly related to the degree of lung hypoplasia, and the mortality rate is approximately 20 per cent.

CASE 79: RECURRENT APNOEAS

History

Baby Carmichael is admitted to the neonatal unit on the day of birth because of a low blood glucose. He was born at 35 weeks' gestation by vaginal delivery after 48 hours of ruptured membranes but an otherwise uneventful pregnancy. His birth weight was 2.0 kg (ninth centile). His mother had two previous pregnancies which resulted in live-born infants. This baby was thought to be jittery within a few hours of birth, and blood glucose was 1.8 mmol/L. A breast-feed was attempted, but he did not latch on well. He was admitted to the neonatal unit at that point for a nasogastric feed, some blood tests were done and the blood glucose rose to 3.2 mmol/L after the first feed. At the age of 6 hours he became apnoeic and a neonatal nurse stimulated him and gave some oxygen. Over the next hour he had five more apnoeic episodes requiring stimulation, and on the last occasion he required a brief period of facemask intermittent positive pressure ventilation.

Examination

Baby Carmichael does not appear dysmorphic, jaundiced or cyanosed. He appears lethargic (reduced spontaneous movement) and his tone feels reduced on handling. Respiratory rate is 50/min with no signs of increased effort, oxygen saturation is 95 per cent in air, and heart rate is 180 beats/min. His temperature is 37.8°C. Femoral pulses, heart sounds and breath sounds are normal. The abdomen is soft with normal bowel sounds. His fontanelle is normotensive. His palate and genitalia are normal.

INVESTIGATIONS		
		Normal
Haemoglobin	17 g/dL	14–22 g/dL
White cell count	21×10^9/L	$10–26 \times 10^9$/L
Platelets	153×10^9/L	$150–400 \times 10^9$/L
C-reactive protein (CRP)	7 mg/L	<5 mg/L
Glucose	3.1 mmol/L	2.8–4.5 mmol/L
Venous blood gas		
pH	7.17	7.35–7.42
Pa_{CO_2}	7.1	4.7–6.0 kPa
Bicarbonate	19	20–26 mmol/L
Base excess	−8.5	+2.5 to −2.5 mmol/L

Questions
- What is the definition of an apnoea?
- What is the most likely reason for the recurrent apnoeas in this baby?
- What additional information about the mother and her treatment would be helpful?
- How should this baby be managed?

ANSWER 79

An apnoea is an episode of cessation of breathing lasting more than 20 s, or a shorter time if there is bradycardia or a colour change. This is distinct from the normal newborn pattern of periodic breathing, where fast respiration alternates with pauses of up to 10 s.

❗ Causes of apnoea in a newborn

- Apnoea of prematurity
- Lung disease, e.g. respiratory distress syndrome
- Congenital heart disease
- Sepsis
- Hypoglycaemia
- Hypothermia
- Sedative drugs (administered to mother in labour, or to baby)
- Neurological insults – cerebral haemorrhage, oedema or seizures
- Anaemia
- Gastro-oesophageal reflux

In this case, the most likely diagnosis is sepsis. The baby was born prematurely after prolonged rupture of membranes – both risk factors for sepsis. He was hypoglycaemic, a common finding in septic newborns, and he has had recurrent and worsening apnoeas. He is lethargic and has a slightly raised temperature. White cell count and CRP are unremarkable, but this is often the case early in the course of neonatal sepsis. The blood gas shows a mixed metabolic and respiratory acidosis, indicating hypoperfusion and hypoventilation. This would be typical of early-onset group B streptococcal (GBS) sepsis.

There is no information provided about whether the mother had any microbiological samples taken, received intrapartum antibiotics, had a fever or had evidence of chorioamnionitis. These are all factors which would affect the risk of sepsis in the newborn. It is also important to know whether the mother received any drugs during labour which may suppress neonatal respiration, e.g. pethidine, or whether she uses any illicit drugs.

Given the presence of two risk factors for early-onset GBS sepsis, if the mother had not received adequate intrapartum antibiotic prophylaxis, the baby should have been assessed, cultures taken and antibiotics commenced at birth. If this was not done as soon as the baby showed the first signs of jitteriness and hypoglycaemia, sepsis should have been suspected. This baby is now in a dangerous situation, where apnoeas may progress to a respiratory arrest. Management priorities are to secure the airway with optimal positioning of the head, ensure adequate breathing with either CPAP or intubation, establish vascular access, give fluid boluses to achieve cardiovascular stability and administer antibiotics as early as possible. After this, further assessment for the source of the sepsis, and to exclude other causes of apnoea, can be undertaken.

 KEY POINTS

- Apnoeas are a final common manifestation of many disease processes in the neonate.
- Any neonate with apnoeas requires prompt evaluation.
- Antibiotics must be administered urgently to a neonate with suspected early-onset sepsis.

CASE 80: A SUDDEN COLLAPSE IN A VENTILATED PRETERM NEONATE

History

A 3-day-old neonate born at 26 weeks gestation, weighing 830 g, is being ventilated on the neonatal intensive care unit. A chest X-ray at 4 hours of age demonstrated severe respiratory distress syndrome. He is being ventilated by conventional mechanical ventilation with pressure settings of 24/3 cmH$_2$O, a ventilator rate of 60 breaths/min and an F_iO$_2$ of 0.55. He has received surfactant and is sedated with an intravenous morphine infusion. His latest arterial gas showed a pH of 7.31, a Po$_2$ of 7.2 kPa and a Pco$_2$ of 6.2 kPa.

Having been very stable over the previous 24 hours, he suddenly deteriorates and becomes deeply cyanosed with an oxygen saturation of 48 per cent. He also becomes bradycardic with a heart rate of 64 beats/min. The nurse immediately puts up the F_iO$_2$ to 0.95 and the oxygen saturation rises to 84 per cent and the heart rate to above 100 beats/min.

Examination

The infant is being hand bagged by the neonatal unit sister with an F_iO$_2$ of 0.95, pressures of 30/4 cmH$_2$O at a rate of approximately 40 breaths/min. The oxygen saturation is 92 per cent. Heart rate is now 170 beats/min. The left hemithorax is moving poorly and auscultation confirms that there is normal air entry on the right but poor air entry on the left. A pneumothorax is suspected. The room lights are lowered and the chest is transilluminated with a fibreoptic cold-light source. The result is inconclusive. Heart sounds are normal and the anterior fontanelle is level. An urgent chest X-ray is ordered (Fig. 80.1) and an arterial blood gas is performed.

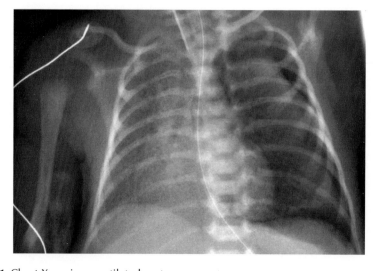

Figure 80.1 Chest X-ray in a ventilated preterm neonate.

INVESTIGATIONS

Arterial gas		Normal
pH	7.22	7.36–7.44
P_{O_2}	6.1 kPa	80–12.0 kPa
P_{CO_2}	7.9 kPa	4.0–6.5 kPa
Base excess	−6.8	(−2.5)–(+2.5) mmol/L

Questions
- What are the causes of a sudden desaturation in a ventilated neonate?
- What is the diagnosis?
- What is the treatment?

ANSWER 80

This question is best answered by considering whether the chest is not moving, whether chest movement is decreased or asymmetrical, or whether chest movement is normal:

- no chest movement
  - ventilator not working or tubing disconnected or kinked
  - endotracheal tube blocked or dislocated
- chest movement decreased or asymmetrical
  - pneumothorax
  - worsening respiratory disease
- chest movement normal
  - right-to-left shunt, e.g. across a patent ductus arteriosus
  - large periventricular haemorrhage
  - severe sepsis.

The diagnosis in this case is a left-sided tension pneumothorax with mediastinal shift to the right (away from the side of the pneumothorax). A chest drain should be inserted immediately.

If a pneumothorax is suspected clinically and cold-light transillumination demonstrates that the chest 'lights up' on that side (the two sides should be compared), this is indicative of a pneumothorax and a chest drain should be inserted and a chest X-ray is unnecessary. If the child deteriorates, a 23g butterfly needle can be inserted into the second intercostal space in the mid-clavicular line. Air can then be aspirated from the pleural space and this can 'buy time' pending the insertion of a chest drain. The largest possible chest drain should be used (usually 8, 10 or 12 FG depending on the size of the infant).

The drain should be inserted above the rib as the intercostal vessels lie immediately below the rib. It should be inserted into the third, fourth or fifth intercostal space in the mid-axillary line. Following insertion and the appropriate connections to an underwater seal, air bubbles should be seen, swinging should be observed on breathing and the infant should rapidly improve. A chest X-ray should be done to ensure that the lung has re-inflated and to check the position of the drain.

 KEY POINTS

- A pneumothorax is a common cause of a sudden deterioration in a ventilated preterm neonate.
- Diagnosis is by cold light transillumination and/or a chest X-ray.
- Urgent treatment is necessary. A needle aspiration can be done in the first instance if the child is very unwell or deteriorating, but definitive treatment is with a chest drain.

History

A baby boy on the postnatal ward starts vomiting at 12 hours of age. The first two vomits consist of milk but subsequent vomits are green-coloured. The infant has not yet passed meconium. The mother was well in pregnancy but the obstetric notes document polyhydramnios. The father has ulcerative colitis and has had multiple operations.

Examination

The boy is apyrexial. His pulse is 196/min, blood pressure 72/35 mmHg and peripheral capillary refill 5 s. His abdomen is not distended. There are no masses, tenderness or organomegaly. There are no other signs.

INVESTIGATIONS		
		Normal
Haemoglobin	18.5 g/dL	14.0–22.0 g/dL
White cell count	27.7 × 10⁹/L	9.0–30.0 × 10⁹/L
Platelets	361 × 10⁹/L	150–400 × 10⁹/L
Sodium	143 mmol/L	135–145 mmol/L
Potassium	5.0 mmol/L	3.5–5.0 mmol/L
Urea	6.2 mmol/L	1.1–4.3 mmol/L
Creatinine	110 μmol/L	27–88 μmol/L
X-ray – see Figure 81.1		

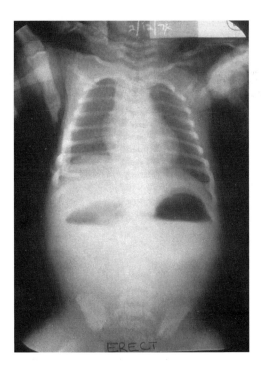

Figure 81.1 X-ray in neonate with bilious vomiting.

Questions

- What does the X-ray show?
- With what condition is this disorder associated?
- What is the treatment?

ANSWER 81

The X-ray demonstrates the classic double bubble appearance due to dilatation of the stomach and the proximal duodenum found in duodenal atresia. It is an erect film which also shows a fluid level in the stomach and duodenum. There is a paucity of gas in the remainder of the abdomen. The polyhydramnios is secondary to the inability of the infant to swallow amniotic fluid (conversely, inability to excrete amniotic fluid in the urine due to renal agenesis or dysgenesis leads to oligohydramnios). As the obstruction is in the upper gastrointestinal tract, there is no abdominal distension.

Down's syndrome is associated with duodenal atresia in 20 per cent of cases. Duodenal atresia is also associated with malrotation, oesophageal atresia and congenital heart disease. Contrast studies are occasionally needed, primarily to rule out malrotation and volvulus.

The pulse rate is raised (normal in a neonate is 100–180 beats/min), the blood pressure is normal and the peripheral capillary refill is prolonged. The urea and creatinine are slightly raised. Initial treatment is with intravenous rehydration to correct the dehydration. A nasogastric tube is inserted and the stomach emptied. Where there is one congenital abnormality, one should look for other abnormalities. Duodenal atresia is associated with heart disease and this needs excluding prior to surgery.

 KEY POINTS

- Bilious vomiting in a newborn should be regarded as a surgical emergency until proven otherwise.
- Duodenal atresia leads to a double bubble appearance on the X-ray.
- There is a strong association with Down's syndrome.

History

Armstrong is a 4-day-old Afro-Caribbean infant who is referred by his midwife to the paediatric day unit because of jaundice. His mother thinks that the jaundice may have commenced within the first 24 hours of life, but she was told by the first midwife that she saw that the baby was fine. The child has also been a little sleepy and has not breast-fed as well as previously. His birth weight was 3.70 kg at term. His mother had a splenectomy after falling off a horse as a teenager. This is her first pregnancy. There is no family history of jaundice.

Examination

The sclera are markedly yellow and the infant is somewhat lethargic. He is well perfused and apyrexial. There is no hepatosplenomegaly and there are no other signs. He weighs 3.40 kg.

INVESTIGATIONS		
		Normal
Haemoglobin	12.1 g/dL	14.0–22.0 g/dL
White cell count	27.7 × 10⁹/L	9.0–30.0 × 10⁹/L
Platelets	361 × 10⁹/L	150–400 × 10⁹/L
Reticulocytes	12 per cent	<2 per cent
Blood film	Occasional spherocytes	
Sodium	143 mmol/L	135–145 mmol/L
Potassium	5.0 mmol/L	3.5–5.0 mmol/L
Urea	6.2 mmol/L	1.1–4.3 mmol/L
Creatinine	110 μmol/L	27–88 μmol/L
Bilirubin	560 μmol/L	<205 μmol/L
Albumin	30 g/L	25–34 g/L
Alanine aminotransferase	48 U/L	6–50 U/L
Alkaline phosphatase	367 U/L	145–420 U/L
C-reactive protein	5 mg/L	<6 mg/L
Baby's blood group	A+	
Maternal blood group	O+	
Direct antiglobulin test (DAT)	Positive	
Glucose-6-phosphate dehydrogenase (G6PD)	7.4 IU/g Hb	4.6–13.5 IU/g Hb
Urine dipstick	No leucocytes or nitrites	

Questions

- What are the causes of jaundice in a neonate?
- Why is neonatal jaundice potentially dangerous?
- What is the cause in this infant?
- What is the treatment?

ANSWER 82

The causes of jaundice are best considered by dividing jaundice into early-onset, normal-onset and late-onset jaundice.

! **Causes of jaundice**

Early onset (first 24 hours, haemolytic jaundice)
- Rhesus haemolytic disease
- ABO incompatibility
- G6PD deficiency (commonest in those of African, Asian, or Mediterranean descent)
- Hereditary spherocytosis

Normal onset
- Physiological (all newborns get a degree of jaundice peaking at 4–5 days)
- Bruising
- Polycythaemia
- Causes of early jaundice

Late onset (>14 days, prolonged jaundice)
- Persistence of a pathological earlier jaundice
- Breast milk jaundice
- Neonatal hepatitis
- Biliary atresia
- Hypothyroidism
- Galactosaemia

Jaundice can also be a non-specific marker of neonatal infection at any stage.

Neonatal jaundice can be dangerous, as unconjugated bilirubin can cross the blood–brain barrier. Very high levels can lead to kernicterus which can cause deafness and choreo-athetoid cerebral palsy.

The cause of the jaundice in this infant is ABO incompatibility. His mother is O+ and will therefore have anti-A and anti-B antibodies in her blood. Theses antibodies can cross the placenta and lead to haemolysis in infants with either blood group A or B. This is further confirmed by the positive DAT (though, on occasion, this test can be negative). The decreased haemoglobin and raised reticulocyte count provide further evidence of haemolysis. The presence of a few spherocytes is common in ABO incompatibility. The normal temperature, normal inflammatory markers and normal urine dipstick make infection unlikely. Unlike Rhesus haemolytic disease, it can occur with the first pregnancy and does not get worse with successive pregnancies.

There are graphs that provide guidelines stating at what bilirubin level treatment with phototherapy and an exchange transfusion are indicated. The guidelines depend on the age of the infant, their weight, gestation and on whether they are well or ill. This infant's bilirubin level is well above the exchange transfusion line. Phototherapy should be commenced immediately and blood taken for cross-match (for O+ blood to minimize further haemolysis). The fall in birth weight of 8 per cent and the raised urea and creatinine suggest a degree of dehydration which could be exacerbating the jaundice.

Maintenance intravenous fluids should therefore be commenced and breast-feeding can be continued. Appropriate lines should be inserted to enable the exchange transfusion to take place. The blood for the transfusion usually has to be ordered from the regional blood transfusion centre. It is possible that the bilirubin will have fallen markedly by the time the blood has arrived, in which case the exchange transfusion may be avoided. Following discharge, the haemoglobin should be monitored, a hearing test arranged and development followed up.

KEY POINTS

- Neonatal jaundice is a potential cause of kernicterus that can lead to deafness and cerebral palsy.
- Jaundice may be more difficult to diagnose in Asian and Afro-Caribbean babies.
- Treatment in severe cases consists of phototherapy ± an exchange transfusion.

CASE 83: A FLOPPY INFANT

History

You are asked to review a baby on the postnatal ward who has not been feeding well. It is a 1-day-old girl, who is the first baby of a 23-year-old Scottish woman. She was born at 39 weeks' gestation and the pregnancy was uncomplicated. The baby was delivered with a ventouse and weighed 3.2 kg (25th–50th centile). The mother reports that the baby has not been very active since she was born and that she has hardly latched on to the breast.

Examination

The baby looks alert and is not dysmorphic. Head circumference is 34.5 cm (50th centile) and the anterior fontanelle is normal. She makes almost no antigravity movements and lies in a 'frog leg' posture. Respiratory, cardiovascular and abdominal examinations are unremarkable. She appears to make conjugate eye movements in all directions, there is no facial asymmetry and she has normal facial expression. Red reflexes are normal. Tone appears to be symmetrically reduced in the upper and lower limbs, and tendon reflexes cannot be elicited. When she is held vertically, she feels like she is slipping downwards, and she is unable to raise her head at all when held horizontally under her abdomen. The sucking reflex is very weak and there appears to be fasciculation of the tongue.

Questions

- What can be concluded from the neurological examination?
- What additional questions should the mother be asked?
- What is the most likely diagnosis and what are the other possible causes of a floppy infant?

ANSWER 83

This baby has a very abnormal neurological examination. The key findings are severe hypotonia and weakness with preservation of facial and eye movements, absent deep tendon reflexes, poor sucking reflex and fasciculation of the tongue. These features indicate a process affecting the lower motor neurones of the entire spinal cord and selective cranial nerve motor nuclei (IX and XII).

In this case it is likely that there is an underlying genetic cause for the baby's condition, so further questions should be asked to try to substantiate this. Parental consanguinity, history of previous pregnancies ending in miscarriage or stillbirth, other family members with medical problems and pregnancies in other family members should be asked about. In the current pregnancy, there may have been reduced fetal movements. The parents should be asked in detail about whether they have any medical problems, and direct questions about symptoms of neuromuscular disease, including weakness, fatiguability and muscle cramps. In assessing any floppy infant, it is important to establish whether an acquired cause may be present, so an assessment should be made of the maternal drug history and of any drugs given during labour, whether any brain or spinal cord injury may have been sustained during delivery, and any risk factors for sepsis or features of metabolic disease.

An infant can be floppy due to 'central' or 'peripheral' (neuromuscular) causes. In the former, deep tendon reflexes are present, and in the latter they are absent and the child has marked weakness. Central causes are much more common than peripheral causes. In this case, the clinical findings are of a peripheral cause and the most likely diagnosis is infantile spinal muscular atrophy (SMA type 1). SMA is an autosomal recessive condition, with type 1 affecting about 1 per 10 000 live births. Sixty per cent of affected infants will be floppy at birth. Motor neurone degeneration leads to progressive weakness and death usually occurs from respiratory complications, e.g. pneumonia, within the first year of life.

! Causes of a floppy infant	
'Central' – hypotonic but not significantly weak	*'Peripheral'– hypotonic, weak, areflexic*
Chromosomal disorder, e.g. Down's syndrome, Prader-Willi syndrome	Infantile spinal muscular atrophy
Brain injury, e.g. hypoxic-ischaemic encephalopathy	Congenital myasthenia
Brain infection or sepsis	Congenital myotonic dystrophy
Metabolic disturbance, e.g. hypoglycaemia	Congenital myopathy
Drug exposure, e.g. pethidine	Congenital muscular dystrophy

🔑 KEY POINTS

- An infant can be floppy due to central or peripheral (neuromuscular) causes.
- Assessment of muscle power and deep tendon reflexes helps to classify the likely causes.
- Central causes of hypotonia are the most common.

CASE 84: A DIFFICULT DELIVERY

History

A 34-year-old woman with gestational diabetes in her first pregnancy is admitted to the labour ward at 41 weeks' gestation in active labour. She is obese (weight 105 kg). Her notes indicate that she was recommended dietary control of her gestational diabetes. Her attendance at antenatal clinic was erratic, and she did not regularly measure her blood glucose concentration. Induction of labour had been discussed previously, as it was felt that the fetus was large. The mother had declined this, stating that she wanted to have a natural birth. The fetal anomaly scan at 20 weeks had been normal, but she had not attended for tests of fetal well-being after 38 weeks' gestation.

The delivery is complicated by severe shoulder dystocia and extra help is summoned, including a neonatal 'crash call'. On arrival of the neonatal team, the baby is still not delivered and the obstetric consultant has just arrived. After 15 min have elapsed from delivery of the head to delivery of the body, a large baby boy is delivered.

Questions
- What immediate problems should be anticipated and why do they occur?
- What will this baby look like at delivery?
- How should the baby be immediately assessed and managed?
- What are the possible complications for the baby?

ANSWER 84

This baby will almost certainly have suffered an acute asphyxial insult as a result of cord compression while delivery of the body was prevented by the shoulder dystocia. The neonatal team should anticipate that the baby will require significant resuscitation and should ensure that a senior neonatologist is present. Obstruction of the fetoplacental circulation for more than a few minutes causes hypoxia, the fetus ceases breathing movements (primary apnoea), becomes bradycardic and circulation is directed to essential organs. Acidosis develops and, after a longer period of asphyxia, episodic reflex gasping occurs. If aeration of the lungs does not occur, these gasps diminish and a phase of terminal apnoea occurs, from which the fetus can only be saved by delivery and artificial ventilation. At delivery this baby will probably be apnoeic, bradycardic or asystolic, pale and floppy.

Resuscitation of the newborn baby is unique. If there has never been aeration of the lungs, this must be achieved before any other interventions will work. The baby should be dried, covered and assessed for colour, tone, breathing and heart rate. If the baby is not breathing, the airway should be opened by placing the head in the neutral position and five inflation breaths should be given. The first few inflation breaths may not produce chest movement because they act to displace lung fluid. The effectiveness of inflation breaths should be assessed by checking for an increase in heart rate. If this has not occurred it should be confirmed that the chest is being inflated before commencing cardiac compressions. This baby may also require adrenaline and sodium bicarbonate to be administered via an emergency umbilical venous catheter in order to achieve a return of cardiac output. The blood glucose should also be checked, especially as his mother had diabetes in pregnancy. After immediate resuscitation, the baby will need to be transferred to the neonatal unit for supportive and neuroprotective care.

The outcome of acute asphyxia can be good if the episode is brief and effective resuscitation is provided. More severe asphyxia can lead to hypoxic-ischaemic encephalopathy (HIE) and death. In addition, shoulder dystocia is associated with brachial plexus injury and fracture of the clavicle and humerus.

 Complications of birth asphyxia

First days after resuscitation	*Long term (mostly after severe HIE)*
Encephalopathy, seizures, cerebral oedema	Cerebral palsy
Hypoventilation	Seizures
Myocardial dysfunction	Sensorineural hearing loss
Persistent fetal circulation	Visual impairment
Renal dysfunction	Learning difficulties
Hypoglycaemia, hyponatraemia	

 KEY POINTS

- If a baby is likely to have suffered severe asphyxia, senior assistance is required.
- Newborn resuscitation has a unique algorithm because the lungs have never been inflated with air.
- Birth asphyxia affects multiple organs, although most long-term complications are neurological.

CASE 85: A NEWBORN WITH CONGENITAL ABNORMALITIES

History

A midwife on the postnatal ward asks for a male infant to be reviewed on the day of birth because she is concerned that his ears look abnormal. The baby was born at term in good condition after a normal vaginal delivery. His mother is a 28-year-old sales manager, and this was her first pregnancy. She received routine antenatal care and her booking blood tests and anomaly scan were unremarkable. She and her partner have no medical problems. She is worried that the baby's ears look abnormal and wants to know whether anything can be done to improve their appearance.

Examination

The birth weight was 2.6 kg (second centile) and head circumference 33.5 cm (ninth centile). The baby has small, abnormal-looking ears and an iris coloboma (a defect in the iris). Respiratory examination is unremarkable. Cardiac examination reveals a heart rate of 140/min, normal femoral pulses, normal apex beat, but a grade 3/6 pansystolic murmur that is loudest at the lower left sternal edge. Abdominal examination reveals a very small penis with undescended testes. Neurological examination is normal, the palate is normal and the hips are normal.

Questions

- What explanation should be given to the parents at this stage?
- What different mechanisms can lead to congenital abnormalities?
- How should a child with multiple congenital abnormalities be assessed?

ANSWER 85

This infant has multiple congenital abnormalities. The explanation given to the parents by the junior doctor must be honest but gentle, and should avoid speculation about prognosis. It would be appropriate to explain that congenital abnormalities are quite common, but in addition to the ear abnormalities the parents have noticed, there are other abnormalities, which need to be assessed by a more senior colleague. The iris coloboma and the genital abnormalities can be pointed out and the heart murmur should be mentioned. The combination of multiple abnormalities suggests an underlying cause or syndrome. The parents will be upset by the news, but will appreciate honesty and hard work in order to give them further information as soon as possible.

Congenital anomalies affect about 3 per cent of live births, although not all of these are obvious at the time of birth. They can be divided into malformations due to errors during morphogenesis, and deformations which affect a previously normally formed part of the fetus. Most malformations do not have a defined aetiology and are considered sporadic.

! **Causes of congenital malformations**

- Genetic
  - chromosomal abnormalities, e.g. 22q11 deletion (DiGeorge syndrome)
  - gene defects, e.g. CHD7 (chromodomain helicase DNA-binding protein 7 mutations causing CHARGE syndrome)
- Environmental
  - maternal factors, e.g. diabetes (cardiac malformations)
  - prescribed drugs, e.g. phenytoin (fetal hydantoin syndrome)
  - recreational drugs, e.g. alcohol (fetal alcohol syndrome)
  - environmental toxins, e.g. dioxins (central nervous system anomalies)
  - infections (e.g. rubella, cytomegalovirus)
- Sporadic

Assessment of a child with multiple congenital abnormalities should determine whether there are other abnormalities, the severity of those already detected, and the underlying cause if possible. Sometimes a characteristic pattern of abnormalities will reveal the diagnosis. Karyotyping should be performed and other specific genetic tests may be required. A clinical geneticist should be asked to assess the child if a unifying diagnosis is not apparent. In this case the findings suggest CHARGE syndrome (coloboma, heart defects, atresia choanae, retardation of growth and development, genital and ear abnormalities). Although there is no respiratory distress, choanal atresia should be excluded (by attempting to pass a nasogastric tube through each nostril). The cardiovascular examination findings would be consistent with a ventricular septal defect, the commonest congenital heart defect. Further assessments by a paediatric cardiologist, ophthalmologist, endocrinologist, urologist, audiological physician and developmental paediatrician will be needed. Making a diagnosis may allow future problems to be anticipated and allows genetic counselling about the recurrence risk in future pregnancies.

 KEY POINTS

- Congenital abnormalities are common.
- If one congenital abnormality is present, you should look for other ones.
- Recognizing a pattern of abnormalities comprising a syndrome is important for prognosis and genetic counselling.

CASE 86: SUDDEN DETERIORATION IN A TERM BABY

History

The midwife finds a 3-day-old male baby on the postnatal ward to be very lethargic and breathing fast. The baby is taken to the neonatal unit for further evaluation. He was born at term by emergency Caesarean section for undiagnosed breech presentation. There was no prolonged rupture of membranes. The pregnancy had been unremarkable to that point and all antenatal scans had been normal. Mother is blood group O-positive, had negative HIV, hepatitis B and syphilis serology and was rubella immune. The delivery was attended by a paediatrician but the baby cried immediately and needed no resuscitation. His birth weight was 3.5 kg (50th centile) and the first-day check was unremarkable. He has been breast-fed and although there were problems latching on initially, he fed well on day 2. He seems rather sleepy and has had frequent non-bilious vomits today. His mother is a 23-year-old woman from Pakistan who speaks good English and this is her first baby.

Examination

The baby's temperature is 36.3°C, his heart rate is 160 beats/min and his respiratory rate is 70 breaths/min. Oxygen saturation is 99 per cent in air, capillary refill is 2–3 s, and blood pressure is 60/40 mmHg. There is subcostal and mild sternal recession. He responds to vigorous stimulation and pain, but otherwise is very lethargic. The chest is clear, heart sounds and femoral pulses are normal, and the abdomen is normal. The fontanelle is normotensive. He has a strong odour which is slightly unpleasant.

INVESTIGATIONS		
		Normal
Venous blood gas analysis		
pH	6.98	7.35–7.42
Pa_{CO_2}	2.62	4.7–6.0 kPa
Base excess	−25.5	+2.5 to −2.5 mmol/L
Lactate	2.1	1.0–1.8 mmol/L
Glucose	5.2	2.2–4.4 mmol/L
Urinalysis		
Glucose	Negative	Negative
Protein	Negative	Negative
Ketones	+++	Negative

Questions

- What are the possible causes of this type of presentation?
- How do you interpret the blood gas analysis?
- What is the most likely cause in this case?
- What is the emergency management?

ANSWER 86

The history describes a term neonate who became very ill over a short period of time. The important diagnoses to consider are discussed in Case 10 (p. 31–32).

! Approach to blood gas interpretation	
	In this case
Look at the pH	pH <7.35, acidosis
Look at the $P\text{CO}_2$	$P\text{CO}_2$ < 4.7 kPa, respiratory compensation
Look at the base excess	Lower than −2.5, metabolic acidosis

The blood gas analysis shows a severe metabolic acidosis, with unsuccessful respiratory compensation. This fits with the clinical picture of a tachypnoeic baby.

Important points to note are the absence of risk factors for sepsis, the absence of signs of circulatory compromise, a lethargic baby with a strong odour, ketonuria and a severe metabolic acidosis without significant hyperlactataemia or hypoglycaemia. These findings point to an inborn error of metabolism, where excess acid is accumulating in the blood due to a metabolic defect. Possible causes include propionic, methylmalonic and isovaleric acidaemias. Remembering the names is less important than recognizing this type of presentation.

Emergency management consists of stopping feeds and starting an infusion of 10 per cent dextrose. Whilst sepsis is unlikely to be the sole cause of the illness, it could be a contributing factor and antibiotics should be administered. The baby needs to be assessed promptly by an experienced paediatrician as he is likely to require intubation and ventilation if he starts to tire or cannot protect his airway. It is likely that sodium bicarbonate would be beneficial to partially correct the acidosis, and the case should be discussed urgently with the regional paediatric metabolic centre, as specific therapies may be recommended even before a certain diagnosis is available. To assist in making a diagnosis, blood should be sent for ammonia, plasma amino acid profile, and urine for amino and organic acid profiles.

This baby had consanguineous parents (first cousins), increasing the risk of an autosomal recessive inborn error of metabolism. He required intubation and ventilation until the acidosis was corrected and he was then transferred to the regional metabolic unit. The diagnosis turned out to be isovaleric acidaemia.

 KEY POINTS

- Metabolic disease can present as a sudden deterioration in the neonatal period.
- Metabolic disease is rare and management must be discussed with an expert.

CASE 87: A CASE OF POSSIBLE TRISOMY 21

History
The midwife on the GP delivery unit has requested a review of a baby born 15 minutes ago. During the baby check she has noted what she thinks are features of trisomy 21 (Down's syndrome). She has looked after the mother for most of the pregnancy. The mother is 26 and the father is 28, and this is their second child – they have an 18-month-old daughter. The pregnancy was unplanned although the parents were delighted when they found out. They had a negative first trimester screen for trisomy 21.

Examination
The baby is a boy with dysmorphic features typical of trisomy 21. Examination of the cardiovascular, respiratory and abdominal systems appears normal.

Questions
- What are the typical dysmorphic features of trisomy 21?
- What specific investigations should this baby have?
- How should you discuss this with the parents?

ANSWER 87

Dysmorphology is the study of human congenital malformations and dysmorphic features are abnormal body characteristics. Some are common in the general population and in isolation are not significant, e.g. single palmar crease. A syndrome is a well-characterized group of such abnormalities occurring together that often point to a single condition as the cause.

! Characteristic dysmorphic features of trisomy 21
• Hypotonia
• Flat face
• Upward slanting palpebral fissures
• Epicanthic folds
• White speckles in the iris (Brushfield spots)
• Short broad hands
• Single palmar and plantar fissures (Simian crease)

There are several associated features, the commonest of which are low IQ (average IQ about 50), congenital heart disease, duodenal atresia and short stature.

Chromosomes must be sent for urgent analysis. This is to confirm the clinical suspicions, look for mosaicism (~1 per cent) that might alter the prognosis and to exclude a translocation. If a translocation is identified, parental chromosomes must be analysed in case one is a carrier with a high risk of recurrence. The incidence of cardiac anomalies is so high (35 per cent) that all children with trisomy 21 should have a cardiac echocardiogram even if no murmur is detected. An atrioventriculoseptal defect (AVSD) is the characteristic association with trisomy 21, but a ventriculoseptal defect is the commonest abnormality.

Although the risk of Down's syndrome rises with maternal age, most mothers of children with Down's syndrome are <30 years as this is the group that has the greatest number of children.

Breaking bad news is never easy but parents will always remember the first discussion. They should be seen by a senior paediatrician with the midwife who knows them well and other family members if they wish. If English is not their first language, an interpreter should be supplied – this should not be a family member as this person needs to be impartial. The discussion should take place in a private room with no phones or bleeps and plenty of time should be allowed. Avoid jargon and use diagrams to help explanations.

It is worth exploring if they have noticed anything. Expect distress, anger, guilt, shame – in fact, any emotion. They are likely to ask how this could happen when they were given a negative screen result. There is a very common misconception amongst the public and professionals that a negative screen completely excludes the diagnosis. Antenatal screening programmes identify those at high risk to whom a definitive diagnostic test (e.g. amniocentesis) should be offered.

Acknowledge that it is normal to forget much of this first meeting. Arrange another meeting soon afterwards and suggest they write down any questions that arise in the meantime. Written material is available from Down's syndrome charities and their websites.

 KEY POINTS

- Negative antenatal screening does not mean zero risk.
- Chromosomes must always be analysed even if the clinical findings are absolutely characteristic of a syndrome.

CASE 88: ABNORMAL MOVEMENTS IN AN 8-DAY-OLD BABY

History

Andrew is an 8-day-old infant referred to the paediatric day unit by the midwife. She and the parents report at least six brief (approximately 30s) episodes of rhythmical shaking of all four limbs associated with abnormal tongue and eye movements. These do not seem to be related to feeds or sleep, nor do they seem to be causing him any distress. Andrew is breast-fed and has regained his birth weight. He was born at term following an uneventful pregnancy to healthy unrelated parents. The delivery was straightforward and Andrew was in good condition at birth. They were discharged home 6 hours after he was born. He is their second baby.

Examination

Andrew looks well. His weight, length and head circumference are all between the 25th and 50th centiles. There are no dysmorphic features. He is afebrile and his pulse is 130 beats/min. Both heart sounds are normal, there are no murmurs and femoral pulses are palpable. Examination of the respiratory and abdominal systems is unremarkable and he has normal male genitalia. His anterior fontanelle is soft. He handles well with normal tone and primitive reflexes. However, during the examination he has two episodes similar to those described by the midwife; both are self-limiting and are accompanied by cyanosis and a change in his cry.

INVESTIGATIONS		
		Normal
Haemoglobin	16.4 g/dL	14.5–22.5 g/dL
White cell count	8.4×10^9/L	$6.0 - 17.5 \times 10^9$/L
Platelets	365×10^9/L	$150–400 \times 10^9$/L
Sodium	138 mmol/L	138–146 mmol/L
Potassium	4.5 mmol/L	3.5–5.0 mol/L
Urea	4.2 mmol/L	1.8–6.4 mol/L
Creatinine	46 µmol/L	27–62 µmol/L
C-reactive protein	<6 g/L	<6 mg/L
Calcium	1.50 mmol/L	2.2–2.7 mmol/L
Phosphate	3.6 mmol/L	1.25–2.10 mmol/L
Alkaline phosphatase (ALP)	305 IU/L	145–420 IU/L
Alanine aminotransferase	28 IU/L	5–45 IU/L
Glucose	4.6 mmol/L	3.3–5.5 mol/L

Questions

- Having witnessed the events during the examination, what should be the immediate management prior to the blood test results?
- Following the blood test results, what further investigations would you request?

ANSWER 88

Andrew is having seizures. Remember these are a symptom, not a diagnosis, and the causes are numerous. The approach to a fitting child is:

1. Give high-flow oxygen, place on a cardiac monitor.
2. Obtain intravenous access. Send relevant tests, starting with the basic and common.
3. Treat immediately what can be treated. Check blood glucose and treat hypoglycaemia after taking specimens to identify a cause. Start intravenous broad-spectrum antibiotics, e.g. benzylpenicillin and gentamicin – although sepsis is unlikely, it is a possibility that needs to be treated.
4. Control the seizures with appropriate anticonvulsants. In neonates this is usually a loading dose of phenobarbital, followed, if necessary, by maintenance.

The results show that Andrew has significant hypocalcaemia, low enough to cause seizures. It is likely to be real because the phosphate is high but, as with all unusual results, it should be repeated. If confirmed, the hypocalcaemia should be treated with intravenous calcium but only after taking samples to investigate the cause. It is crucial not to lose this opportunity to make a diagnosis because endocrine and metabolic pathways correct very rapidly.

> **! Causes of hypocalcaemia in infancy**
>
> - Prematurity
> - Hypoxic ischaemic encephalopathy (HIE)
> - Hypoparathyroidism – transient (associated with prematurity, HIE or maternal diabetes) or permanent
> - Hypomagnesaemia – magnesium facilitates release of parathormone (PTH)
> - Exchange transfusion – citrate in transfused blood chelates calcium to prevent clotting
> - Familial activating mutations of the calcium-sensing receptor – the calcium level at which PTH is released is lower than normal; some cases labelled as 'familial hypoparathyroidism' are probably this disorder
> - Maternal hypercalcaemia – suppresses fetal PTH
> - Maternal vitamin D deficiency
> - In older children, vitamin D deficiency is the commonest cause, but the ALP would be high due to the increased bone turnover in rickets (see Case 22, p. 66).

Most of these can be excluded from the history. The next tests to send are magnesium, parathyroid hormone (PTH), vitamin D and maternal bone biochemistry. However, the high phosphate (PTH is phosphaturic) and normal ALP suggest hypoparathyroidism. The causes of permanent hypoparathyroidism that present in the neonatal period include DiGeorge syndrome – a disorder associated with microdeletions of chromosome 22q11.2, congenital heart disease and thymic aplasia. PTH is not available therapeutically so treatment of hypoparathyoidism is with vitamin D, but this does not stop the renal loss of calcium that PTH normally prevents. To minimize the risk of nephrocalcinosis, calcium is maintained at low normal or mildly subnormal levels and the urinary calcium/ creatinine ratio is monitored.

All children with neonatal seizures of any cause are at risk of developmental problems and need surveillance.

 KEY POINTS

- In any case of hypocalcaemia or hypoglycaemia, relevant samples should be taken before treatment to maximize the opportunity of making a definitive diagnosis.
- Children with neonatal seizures of any cause are at risk of developmental problems and need surveillance.

MISCELLANEOUS

CASE 89: A FRACTURE IN AN INFANT

History

Bobby is a 13-week-old baby brought to the A&E department one evening by his parents because he is not moving his left leg. They both report that he seemed fine during his bath the previous evening and went to bed as usual. He was awake on and off during the evening, but with a recent cold has been more difficult to settle. They share the baby's care and last night it was his father's turn, but he is adamant that he noticed nothing untoward when he fed him and changed his nappy. Bobby's mother recalls being woken by him crying but is not sure of the time. They both noticed the leg when they woke up this morning. Bobby's mother wanted to bring him in straight away but his father persuaded her that it was probably the way he had slept and that they should wait a while.

Bobby was born at 37 weeks. He was in good condition at birth and they have no concerns about his development. He has been bottle-fed from birth and is often difficult to feed, with quite severe symptoms of gastro-oesophageal reflux. The GP has prescribed Gaviscon but without much improvement. He is on no other regular medication. No diseases run in the family. His father is aged 19 and his mother is 18. They recently moved from a more rural area in the hope of finding employment but with no success yet. Neither of them has any family locally nor has anyone else taken care of Bobby in the past couple of days. They are living in a two-room flat and the baby sleeps in a cot in their bedroom.

Examination

Bobby is a healthy, well-grown baby. The parent-held record shows that he has been gaining weight along the 9th centile. His length is on the 25th centile, as is his head circumference. The only abnormality is that he is not moving his left leg and cries in pain when it is moved. There is soft tissue swelling overlying the left femur. His temperature is 37.7°C and he is a bit coryzal. His sclerae are normal.

 INVESTIGATIONS

An X-ray of Bobby's left leg is shown in Figure 89.1.

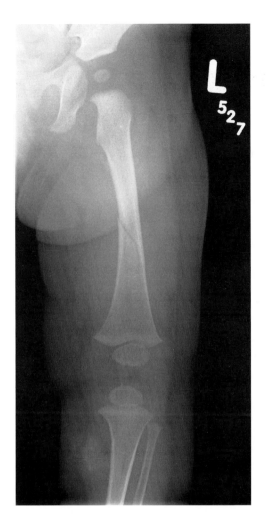

Figure 89.1 An X-ray of Bobby's left leg.

Questions
- What does the X-ray show?
- What are the worrying features in the history?
- What other investigations must he have?
- Outline the management

ANSWER 89

The X-ray shows a mid-shaft spiral fracture of the left femur. The majority of childhood fractures are accidental with an explanation that fits the injury. However, non-accidental injury (NAI) must always be considered and there are certain patterns of presentation and findings that ring alarm bells. The child's age and mobility are very important factors. The fracture site and type are also important. Metaphyseal and posterior rib fractures are very suspicious and a spiral fracture suggests a twisting injury – unlikely in a non-weight-bearing infant. So the most worrying features in this history are an unexplained spiral long bone fracture in an infant who is immobile and under constant adult supervision. There has also been a delay in reporting the injury. All of these are features that make any injury more likely to be non-accidental. Others include:

- a history that is not consistent with the injury
- a history that changes with time
- inappropriate reaction(s) of carer(s) – vague, elusive or aggressive
- history of a suspicious injury or NAI in child and/or siblings.

Any infant with suspected NAI must have a full skeletal survey with an expert radiology assessment because not all fractures are detectable clinically. Rib fractures may be inconspicuous initially and a bone scan and/or a repeat chest X-ray may also be needed. These investigations should also help exclude the rare differential of osteogenesis imperfecta. He should also have a brain CT scan to exclude injuries such as a subdural haemorrhage. If there is bruising, a full blood count and a clotting screen are necessary.

! **Steps in management**

- Admit to manage the fracture and as a place of safety
- Pain relief and immobilization in traction
- Check the child protection register
- Document, date and sign the history, examination and investigations
- Inform a senior paediatrician, who will confirm the findings and explain openly and non-judgmentally why there are concerns, what is going to happen next and who will be involved
- Refer immediately to Social Care. Where appropriate, they will involve the police
- Attend the multidisciplinary child protection conference to which the parents are invited. Information is shared between all professional groups. Outcomes are the decision of the conference, not of individuals. The aim is always to act in the child's best interest

---

This family have other risk factors for NAI. They are young, have no local support, and there have been difficulties with feeding. The father admitted to losing his temper in the middle of the night after neighbours complained about the crying. He wrenched the baby's leg trying to get it out of his sleep suit.

 KEY POINTS

- The possibility of non-accidental injury should be considered in any childhood fracture.
- Thorough documentation is vital in all possible cases of non-accidental injury.
- Communication between all professional groups is essential in deciding the outcome for the child and family.

CASE 90: A VAGINAL DISCHARGE

History

Jasmine is a 4-year-old girl who presents to her GP with a yellow smelly vaginal discharge. Her mother states that her daughter is itching a lot and occasionally finds it difficult and painful to pass urine. There is no history of a foreign body. She is otherwise well. A week previously she and her two siblings all had a cold. She has never had a urinary tract infection. She had her tonsils and adenoids removed last year. Her mother has type 1 diabetes and hypothyroidism.

Examination

She is apyrexial. Her blood pressure 104/70 mmHg. There are no abdominal signs. The vulval and perianal areas look erythematous with scratch marks and some areas of linear ulceration. A yellowish discharge can be seen. There is no bruising.

INVESTIGATIONS
Vulval swab – numerous white blood cells (WBCs), haemolytic *Streptococcus* grown Urine microscopy, culture and sensitivity (M, C+S) – numerous white blood cells, mixed growth of three organisms

Questions

- What is the likely diagnosis?
- What is the differential diagnosis?
- What is the treatment?

ANSWER 90

The likely diagnosis is vulvovaginitis. Prepubertal girls may have a clear sticky discharge that resolves with menarche. However, a malodorous discharge indicates pathology. It is most likely that a *Streptococcus* was the cause of the upper respiratory tract infection and that this infection was transmitted to the genital area by the child's fingers. It is not uncommon to get a degree of dysuria in association with vulvovaginitis. Occasionally vaginal bleeding may occur. To definitively diagnose a urinary tract infection, there has to be a pure growth of 10^5 colony-forming units/mL $\pm$ WBCs. Jasmine's results do not fulfil this criteria. Poor perineal hygiene may cause or exacerbate vulvovaginitis, which often presents shortly after girls have started self-toileting. Masturbation may also lead to vulvovaginitis. Pinworms may be associated with perianal itching, especially at night, and in about 20 per cent of cases there is an associated vulvovaginitis. If no worms are visible, Sellotape can be applied to the perianal skin, stuck onto a glass slide and then sent for microscopy to look for enterobius ova. Herpes infection can also lead to vulvovaginitis. It leads to vesicles and to discrete ulcers. These are usually due to digital contact with cold sores, but the possibility of sexual abuse should also be borne in mind. Viral swabs should be taken. Recurrent vulvovaginitis usually ceases at puberty.

The differential consists of candidal infection, a foreign body, sexually transmitted disease and the very rare botryoid sarcoma. Candida leads to a creamy white discharge, vulval itching and dysuria. It is rare prepubertally but may occur in diabetics or following antibiotic use. A foreign body may consist of toilet paper or a toy. In young children it may be visible on inspection, but on occasion may require an examination under anaesthetic. Evidence of infection with an organism such as chlamydia or gonorrhoea suggests sexual abuse and should prompt a child protection investigation. A sarcoma usually presents with a bloodstained vaginal discharge. On examination, a fleshy haemorrhagic lesion is seen, which is often described as 'grape-like'.

Treatment consists of a 1-week course of penicillin. Basic hygiene measures should also be advocated, such as cleaning oneself from front to back after a bowel motion, using loose-fitting cotton knickers, having daily baths or showers using simple soaps (avoiding bubble baths or other irritants) and allowing air to dry. A short course of topical oestrogen cream may also be helpful.

 KEY POINTS

- Vulvovaginitis is common in prepubertal girls.
- Advice on hygiene $\pm$ antibiotics is effective in treating this condition.
- In children with a vaginal discharge, the possibility of sexual abuse should also be considered.

CASE 91: AN ODD SHAPED HEAD

History
Colin is a 5-month-old boy who is referred to the paediatric clinic by his GP for assessment of an abnormal head shape. He was born at 38 weeks' gestation by forceps delivery. Apart from a small bruise across his forehead, no abnormality was noted at that time. He has not had any medical problems since birth, but his parents have noted that over the last few months his head shape has become increasingly asymmetrical. They are very worried about this cosmetically, and the GP has worried them further by suggesting that he may have craniosynostosis. Colin is the first child of American parents who both work in banking. He was bottle-fed from birth because his mother found breast-feeding very difficult. He is described as a contented child who sleeps well and cries little. Developmental history reveals that he can sit with support from cushions, although he prefers lying on his back, he can pick up objects with the palm of either hand and puts them in his mouth, he holds his milk bottle, he enjoys vocal turn-taking and makes a range of sounds. When he was younger, he mainly lay on the right side of his head, but this is less obvious now as he is able to move about more.

Examination
Colin is a healthy-looking boy. His weight is 7.5 kg (50th centile), his length is 67 cm (75th centile) and his head circumference is 43.5 cm (50th centile). His head is parallelogram-shaped when viewed from above, with the right occipital region appearing flattened (see Fig. 91.1). There is no ridging over any of the cranial sutures. His face appears symmetrical and there are no dysmorphic features. He does not have a squint and cranial nerve function appears normal. His anterior fontanelle is normal.

Questions
- What is the most likely cause of the abnormal head shape?
- What is craniosynostosis and what complications can it cause?
- What treatment might be available for Colin?

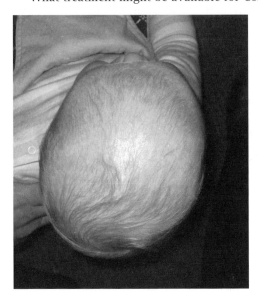

Figure 91.1 Colin's head shape. (Reproduced with permission of The London Orthotic Consultancy Ltd.)

ANSWER 91

Colin almost certainly has positional (deformational) plagiocephaly. This occurs when asymmetrical pressure on the developing occiput or skull base results in oblique flattening of the posterior skull. Causes include an asymmetrical sleeping position, torticollis and cervical spine abnormalities. There may be an underlying reason why the child sleeps in an asymmetrical position, such as a neuromuscular disorder. The typical history of positional plagiocephaly is that the baby either is born with or develops an abnormal head shape sometime after birth, which then improves with time. If the child is born with the abnormality, the deformation is due to compression *in utero*. As mobility increases, the likelihood of persistent asymmetrical pressure decreases, and in most cases head shape will return to normal. The major differential diagnosis is craniosynostosis. The incidence of positional posterior plagiocephaly increased markedly following campaigns to encourage infants to sleep on their back to reduce the risk of sudden infant death.

Craniosynostosis is premature fusion of one or more sutures of the skull, resulting in an abnormal skull shape. The deformity is often present at birth, is progressive and does not improve spontaneously. It can result in raised intracranial pressure and developmental delay. The head shape depends on the involved suture(s). For example, sagittal synostosis results in a narrow head with an enlarged anteroposterior dimension, while lambdoid synostosis results in occipital plagiocephaly. Superficially, the head shape in lambdoid synostosis may be thought to be similar to that in positional plagiocephaly, but in fact there are important differences in the way the structure of the skull and face change, which can be used to make a diagnosis. In positional plagiocephaly, the fontanelle retains a diamond shape. Looking down on the top of the head, the head shape is a parallelogram in positional plagiocephaly, produced by unilateral flattening of the occipital area with ipsilateral bossing of the frontal and parietal bones. In lambdoid synostosis, there is unilateral flattening of the occiput but less frontal asymmetry, resulting in a rhomboid head shape. In positional plagiocephaly, the ear ipsilateral to the flattened occiput is displaced anteriorly, while in lambdoid synostosis it is displaced posteriorly and inferiorly. In craniosynostosis, a ridge is often palpable in the area of the fused suture. Where doubt remains, a skull X-ray or CT scan can be used to further assess the sutures and craniofacial structure. Sometimes craniosynostosis is part of a syndrome such as Apert's or Crouzon's syndrome, where the associated facial and other abnormalities usually make the diagnosis obvious.

It is likely that Colin's head shape will improve spontaneously, and even if it does not completely return to normal, hair growth will disguise much of the abnormal appearance. If the problem is severe or continues to worsen then treatment may be indicated. Helmet moulding may have some benefit by rebalancing growth of the skull. In the most severe cases, surgical intervention is sometimes warranted.

 KEY POINTS

- Positional posterior plagiocephaly is the most common cause of abnormal head shape.
- Craniosynostosis usually causes progressive deformation with a ridge palpable over the fused suture(s).
- Positional plagiocephaly usually improves spontaneously.

CASE 92: A DROWSY TODDLER

History

Jonathan is a 21-month-old boy referred to the paediatric day unit by his GP. He was seen in the surgery the previous day with diarrhoea and vomiting and seemed to have tummy ache. The vomit contained a small amount of fresh blood, but as he was otherwise well and cardiovascularly stable, admission had been deferred because his mother is 36 weeks into her fourth pregnancy. Instead, later that day, the GP rang to check how he was and was reassured to hear that he seemed to have recovered and was tolerating drinks and some food. However, this morning he seems lethargic and a finger-prick blood glucose test performed by his GP was only 3.1 mmol/L. Jonathan is the youngest of three children, the older two being 6 and 3 years old. His father is in the navy and is currently at sea.

Examination

He looks unwell. His airway is patent, his respiratory rate is 26 breaths/min and his pulse rate is 180 beats/min with a capillary refill time of 5 s. His blood pressure is 60/35 mmHg. He is jaundiced. Both heart sounds are present and normal. Examination of the respiratory and abdominal systems is normal. He is drowsy but knows his mother and responds to her voice. He resists examination and withdraws to pain. There is no meningism and there are no focal neurological signs.

INVESTIGATIONS		
		Normal
Haemoglobin	12.3 g/dL	11.5–15.5 g/dL
White cell count	8.4×10^9/L	$6.0-17.5 \times 10^9$/L
Platelets	140×10^9/L	$150-400 \times 10^9$/L
Prothrombin time	19 s	11–15 s
Partial thromboplastin time	32 s	25–35 s
Sodium	138 mmol/L	138–146 mmol/L
Potassium	3.6 mmol/L	3.5–5.0 mmol/L
Urea	8.2 mmol/L	1.8–6.4 mmol/L
Creatinine	33 μmol/L	27–62 μmol/L
Glucose	2.9 mmol/L	3.3–5.5 mmol/L
Bilirubin	85 mmol/L	2–26 mmol/L
Alanine aminotransferase (ALT)	1875 IU/L	5–45 IU/L
Alkaline phosphatase	2624 IU/L	145–420 IU/L
Albumin	32 g/L	39–50 g/L
C-reactive protein	<6 mg/L	<6 mg/L
Lactate	3.2	0.8–1.5 mmol/L
Venous blood gas on 15 L/min of oxygen		
pH	7.28	7.35–7.45
P_{CO_2}	3.8 kPa	4.5–6.0 kPa
Bicarbonate	17 mmol/L	22–29 mmol/L

Questions

- What pathological processes are evident from his clinical signs and investigations?
- What is the most likely unifying cause?
- How is this condition managed?

ANSWER 92

Firstly, this boy has acute liver dysfunction. He has a prolonged prothrombin time, hypoglycaemia and low albumin – these are markers of the manufacturing processes of the liver. There is liver inflammation with an elevated ALT and bilirubin. Secondly, he has clinical and biochemical evidence of tissue underperfusion and increased anaerobic metabolism. He has a tachycardia, borderline hypotension and a prolonged capillary refill time with a metabolic acidosis and a high lactate. There is a compensatory reduction in the Pco_2 (see Case 86, p. 253). Thirdly, there are clinical symptoms and signs suggestive of mild encephalopathy, although his drowsiness could be due to the hypoglycaemia. Finally, note the high urea. This could be due to dehydration but his diarrhoea and vomiting were resolving and the creatinine is normal. It is more likely to be due to the digestion of blood following upper gastrointestinal tract bleeding. Ask about melaena stools.

The most likely unifying cause is some form of poisoning. This history is classical for iron toxicity. Iron is corrosive to the gastrointestinal mucosa, causing abdominal pain, nausea, vomiting and diarrhoea within a few hours of ingestion with haematemesis and bloody diarrhoea in more severe toxicity. Thereafter, there is an interlude with an apparent recovery from about 8–16 hours. This boy has entered the third stage (16–24 hours) with progressive systemic involvement due to the vasodilator effects of iron and mitochondrial poisoning. Toxicity is related to the amount of ferrous iron ingested, which varies according to the particular iron salt. All preparations carry this information, e.g. a ferrous fumarate tablet 210 mg contains 65 mg of ferrous iron. Toxicity is unlikely if <20 mg/kg is ingested but the risk increases steadily thereafter. Not many tablets are needed to cause significant poisoning.

! Management of iron poisoning

- Give oxygen and intravenous fluids to manage poor perfusion
- Treat hypoglycaemia
- Send the family home to check for missing drugs and to bring in any remaining drugs for identification
- Whole iron tablets are radio-opaque – an abdominal X-ray to confirm ingestion may help
- Try to remove the poison. If taken within 1 hour of presentation or tablets visible in stomach on X-ray, consider gastric lavage with a wide-bore tube
- Measure serum iron urgently, but remember that it may be spuriously low if taken > 8 hours post-ingestion
- Try to estimate the quantity of iron ingested and the risk of toxicity
- Discuss with National Poisons Information Service (24 hour service) who will advise about treatment with desferrioxamine, a specific chelator of iron
- Discuss with a specialist liver unit

This child's mother was receiving iron treatment during her pregnancy and found the pack in his bedroom. Iron is one of the most common causes of childhood accidental poisoning because iron-containing preparations are widely available and often resemble sweets. Some units ask a health visitor to undertake a home visit after any case of accidental poisoning to assess overall home safety and to remind parents about keeping all drugs out of reach of children.

KEY POINTS

- Advice should be sought from the National Poisons Information Service if there is any doubt about the management of a case of poisoning.
- Iron is one of the most common causes of childhood poisoning.

History

Jake is a 13-year-old boy referred to the A&E department by his GP with a sudden change in behaviour. The previous day he complained of tiredness, but had been playing a lot of football with his friends and training at a club. He watched television during the evening and apparently slept well. The morning of the admission he had been quieter than usual but had gone to school. His mother was phoned to say that his behaviour was very out of character; he was refusing to obey commands and looked 'spaced out'. At home Jake seemed unable to perform simple tasks such as changing his clothes, putting on his pyjamas rather than his shorts. He then became rather jumpy and nervous. He denies any headache and there have been no abnormal movements witnessed. He has had no diarrhoea or vomiting. Jake has no significant past medical history. His older brother has epilepsy, which is well controlled with lamotrigine. Jake struggles at school, needing extra help with literacy and maths. There were some minor behaviour problems in his junior school but nothing since.

Examination

Jake looks generally well. His height is on the 91st centile and his weight is on the 75th centile. He is afebrile. His pulse is 88 beats/min and his blood pressure is 110/75 mmHg. Examination of the cardiovascular, respiratory and abdominal systems is unremarkable. There is no meningism. When asked, he does not know the day of the week, which town the hospital is in, or his birthday. He cannot remember the name of his favourite football club. He becomes agitated and aggressive when being questioned and is very slow to answer. Both pupils appear dilated and have a slightly sluggish response to light. He is uncooperative with attempts at fundoscopy. There are no obvious focal neurological signs but he cannot understand the instructions for the tests of cerebellar function, e.g. finger–nose test. His gait is normal.

Questions
- What further history should you specifically obtain?
- What other investigations would you request and why?

ANSWER 93

This previously healthy teenage boy has developed an acute confusional state. One of the most obvious causes is drug ingestion, either recreational or a deliberate overdose, possibly with his brother's lamotrigine. It is important to ask the family specific questions. Has he been out of their sight? Are there any other drugs in the house? If necessary, send them home to check and make sure none are missing. Phone the school and his friends. All these steps could be life-saving. A urine screen for 'drugs of abuse' and toxicology, including lamotrigine, should be requested but the result will take some time.

However, never jump to conclusions – there are numerous other possibilities. With an acute history, metabolic problems are unlikely although they must be excluded. Hyponatraemia could be due to inappropriate antidiuretic hormone secretion following an unreported head injury. Hypercalcaemia and renal failure are likely to have a more insidious onset and other symptoms, such as tiredness. Thyroid disease is a possibility. Thyrotoxicosis can present with an isolated behaviour disturbance such as school phobia. At this age, a previously undiagnosed inborn error of metabolism is unlikely but is certainly possible, especially in a child with learning difficulties. Measure blood sugar (bedside and laboratory), a venous pH, lactate and ammonia. Keep urine for amino and organic acid analysis. Ask the laboratory to keep any spare blood in case it is needed for future analysis. Most will do so for up to 6 months.

Even in the absence of clinical signs, bacterial and viral infections are possible diagnoses. They are also treatable. Send a full blood count, C-reactive protein, blood cultures, a midstream urine and acute viral titres. If indicated, convalescent titres can be sent 10–14 days later. It is safest to start treatment with broad-spectrum antibiotics, e.g. cefotaxime, and aciclovir. A lumbar puncture is currently contraindicated because he is very confused and raised intracranial pressure cannot be excluded. It may be indicated once he has improved.

An acute neurological event must also be excluded, including seizures and migraine. He merits an urgent CT and/or a MRI scan and an EEG.

This boy's EEG the following day showed generalized bursts of spike and slow-wave activity with a frontotemporal emphasis. He recovered within 24 hours but went on to have further similar episodes of confusion, culminating in a generalized seizure. The final diagnosis was complex partial epilepsy with secondary generalization. He responded very well to anticonvulsants.

 KEY POINTS

- Do everything possible to identify any drug that a child might have taken inadvertently or deliberately. It might save their life.
- Never assume that an acute confusional state is due to drug ingestion at any age.

History

Laura is a 14-year-old girl who is admitted to the A&E department. Her friend who accompanies her states that she collapsed on the pavement having had a bottle of vodka and then disappears. She has vomited once in the ambulance and once in casualty. There is no other history available. Her parents are not present.

Examination

Airway, breathing and circulation are stable. Glasgow Coma Score (GCS) is 6. Temperature is 36.4°C. There are no signs of trauma, no focal neurological signs and no other signs.

INVESTIGATIONS	
Urea and electrolytes	Normal
Bone chemistry	Normal
Liver function tests	Normal
Blood glucose	5.6 mmol/L
Blood alcohol level	210 mg/100 mL.

Questions

- Should this child be ventilated?
- What other investigation should be performed?
- What treatment should be administered?
- What wider aspects of this adolescent's case should be looked into?

ANSWER 94

The airway of any child with a GCS of 8 or less is at risk. An anaesthetist should be called urgently to monitor the airway and breathing. A blood gas may help the assessment. Most children in this setting will manage without being intubated and slowly, spontaneously recover.

A cranial computed tomography (CT) scan should be done. There is very little history. Although there are no external marks of a head injury or focal neurological signs, it is possible that Laura sustained a head injury when she fell on the pavement and that this partly accounts for her low GCS. The vomiting is probably secondary to the alcohol ingestion but may be secondary to a head injury.

Maintenance intravenous fluids (5 per cent dextrose/0.45 per cent saline) should be administered to help avoid the hangover headache that is primarily due to dehydration. Hourly GCS observations should be performed.

Binge-drinking is very common in teenagers. It is important to try to find out the child's name and contact their family as soon as possible. Social services should be contacted to inform them of what has happened and to find out if she is known to them. When she is awake it would be worth asking whether she takes recreational drugs and consider doing urine toxicology, if appropriate. One should also ask about the possibility of sexual abuse whilst she was drunk and unconscious. However, if there are no allegations of sexual abuse and no evidence to suggest it (e.g. missing or torn knickers) then this need not be pursued. If there are concerns about the possibility of sexual abuse, a forensic medical examiner should be contacted to do the necessary examination and to take the necessary forensic swabs. There is an association between alcohol abuse, behavioural disorders and depression. In some cases, psychiatric and/or social work input and follow-up is required.

 KEY POINTS

- Binge-drinking is very common in adolescents.
- In drunken teenagers, always measure the blood glucose level.
- In children with a diminished GCS, a cranial CT should be done to rule out the possibility of a coexisting intracranial injury.
- Remember to consider the psychosocial aspects of the case.

History

Amy is a 3-year-old girl brought to the GP by her mother. Her health visitor has discussed her previously in the surgery and has been trying to persuade Amy's mother to attend. She is worried about Amy's behaviour, although Amy's mother laughs it off and thinks that it is just a phase she is going through. Amy has a long-standing habit of licking and chewing objects such as toys, and picking plaster and paint off walls and eating it. This will happen anywhere, including paint from shop windows. As a toddler she also used to eat mud and stones but this has recently reduced. Her mother reports some complaints of tummy ache and constipation but is otherwise not worried about her daughter.

Examination

Amy immediately starts exploring the surgery climbing onto the couch and windowsill before the GP stops her. She tips out the waste bin and starts to rummage through the contents and nibble paper towels. She also turns the taps on and off, splashing water over the floor. Her mother seems oblivious to all this and is seeking a letter about re-housing. From time to time during the consultation, Amy comes to the GP and reaches out to be picked up and sits on her knee for a while being cuddled. The GP notices that Amy's fingers, nails and clothes are dirty and she has head lice. The health visitor has been monitoring her height and weight, and although her weight has been following the 2nd centile and her height is just above it, she is below the target range for her parents (25th–75th). On examination she is anaemic and looks thin but there are no other signs.

INVESTIGATIONS		
	Normal	
Haemoglobin	9.3 g/dL	11.5–15.5 g/dL
White cell count	8.4×10^9/L	6.0–17.5×10^9/L
Platelets	365×10^9/L	150–400×10^9/L
Mean cell volume	56 fL	77–95 fL
Mean corpuscular haemoglobin	20 pg	24–30 pg
Blood film – microcytic, hypochromic, with basophilic stippling		

Questions

- What is the diagnosis?
- What further information should you gather?
- What complications have arisen?
- What is the management?

ANSWER 95

Amy has pica, the repeated or chronic ingestion of non-nutritive substances. This is almost universal in infants and toddlers but abnormal after the age of 2 years and needs investigation.

It is very unusual for a child to spontaneously reach out to a relatively unknown adult for comfort. This behaviour should always raise the possibility of emotional and social neglect and these are known predisposing factors for pica. Others include autism and learning difficulties and the GP needs to ensure that there is no significant developmental delay. Her social behaviour is not typical of autism. The difficulty persuading the mother to attend, her indifference to the problem and her behaviour during the consultation all add to the concerns. Amy is also small for her family and thin. Emotional and physical neglect can lead to psychosocial dwarfism. A full social history should be gathered about the family and their circumstances. Who else is at home? Does the mother have a partner and is he the father of Amy? Is there a history of drug or alcohol abuse or domestic violence? Are there other children? Is this family known to Social Care?

Anaemia and lead poisoning have developed. The microcytic, hypochromic anaemia is strongly indicative of iron deficiency, which is common in childhood and almost always dietary in origin. It is even more common in pica. Basophilic stippling is characteristic of lead poisoning, another known complication of pica. Sources include lead-containing paint from both buildings and imported painted toys. Symptoms range from colicky abdominal pain and constipation to headache, drowsiness, fits and coma in lead encephalopathy. Once in the intestine, lead competes with iron and calcium for binding sites, so if either or both of these are deficient, lead absorption is enhanced. Hyperactivity, as in this case, is frequently a manifestation of lead poisoning in pre-school and young school-aged children.

The management of this child has two components, medical and psychosocial:

- *Medical management*
  - urgent referral to hospital
  - exclude other causes for poor growth and weight gain, e.g. coeliac disease
  - measure blood lead and seek advice from the National Poisons Information Service about the need for chelating agents
  - check blood ferritin and a haemoglobinopathy screen and give a 3-month course of iron
  - measure bone biochemistry and vitamin D and consider treatment with vitamin D or a multivitamin preparation to minimize lead absorption
- *Psychosocial management*
  - referral to Social Care for a multidisciplinary assessment of the whole family
  - try to establish the source of lead and remove it or restrict access to it – involve the Health Protection Agency
  - likely to need referral to Child and Family Therapy service for behaviour management.

KEY POINTS

- Exclude lead poisoning in any child with a history of pica.
- In lead poisoning, investigate and treat any coexisting calcium and iron deficiency to minimize lead absorption.
- Emotional and social neglect are known predisposing factors for pica.

History

Gregory is a 5-year-old boy who has been brought to the A&E department by ambulance after a friend's parent dialled 999. While at their son's birthday party he complained of tummy ache, started vomiting and then had profuse watery diarrhoea. He also became acutely wheezy and was struggling to breathe. His voice became hoarse and he was obviously scared. The ambulance crew report that when they arrived he was barely conscious, had severe stridor and markedly increased work of breathing. He is known to have asthma and eczema, both reasonably well controlled. His parents report that he had cow's milk intolerance as a toddler, with vomiting and poor weight gain, and develops urticaria if he eats eggs. However, he has never had anything like this before.

Examination

Gregory is sitting up on the trolley with a salbutamol nebulizer in progress. There is obvious stridor with tracheal tug. His work of breathing is increased with subcostal and intercostal recession and he is using his accessory muscles of respiration. He is quiet but can say his name. His oxygen saturation is 92 per cent. His pulse is 160/min and his capillary refill time is 4 s. His heart sounds are normal. There is widespread expiratory wheeze. Abdominal examination is normal. He is flushed and his lips and face are swollen. He has widespread urticaria.

Questions

- The ambulance crew gave him life-saving drug treatment. What was it?
- How would you continue his immediate management?
- Once he has recovered, what investigations would you undertake?

ANSWER 96

Gregory has had an acute anaphylactic reaction – presumably to something he ate at the party. The emergency drug treatment of anaphylactic shock is intramuscular 1/1000 (1 mg/mL) adrenaline (see Table 96.1). All health care professionals involved in procedures that could cause anaphylaxis, e.g. practice nurses giving immunizations, are trained to give this as first line. They do not need to wait for a doctor's prescription.

Table 96.1 Dose of intramuscular adrenaline (epinephrine) for anaphylactic shock (UK Resuscitation Council)

Age	Dose (µg)	Volume (mL) 1/1000 adrenaline
Under 6 months	50	0.05
6 months–6years	120	0.12
6–12 years	250	0.25
12–18 years	500	0.5

The management of acute anaphylaxis is essentially 'ABC' – airway, breathing, circulation. Oxygen should be administered at all times. The stridor is evidence of upper airway obstruction and the wheeze indicates lower airway obstruction. If the stridor and respiratory distress are severe, he should receive nebulized adrenaline, repeated if necessary. If the stridor does not improve, the anaesthetist should be called. In severe cases, an ENT surgeon will also be required. Intravenous hydrocortisone will also help the stridor and wheezing but may take a few hours to work. Nebulized salbutamol should be continued as necessary to treat the acute bronchoconstriction. He is flushed and has urticaria and is therefore peripherally vasodilated. His capillary refill time is prolonged. His blood pressure should be measured. He should receive a 20 mL/kg bolus of intravenous 0.9 per cent saline plus a dose of antihistamine, e.g. chlorpheniramine.

Once he is stable, further history should be obtained to try and identify the culprit food. Skin-prick tests and/or total IgE and RAST (radioallergosorbent test) to specific foods should be requested (but these need to be done a week or more after the last administration of an antihistamine or steroid). Peanuts and nuts are hidden in many foodstuffs and would be high on the list. Lifelong exclusion is required but inadvertent ingestion is a risk. He will need to have available at all times a pack for self (or carer) administration of intramuscular adrenaline from a pre-assembled syringe and needle, e.g. Epipen. Most importantly his family need advance instruction on how to use it. They should also have a supply of oral antihistamine.

If he is found to be allergic to a specific food he will need referral to a dietician for specialist advice. Self-administered adrenaline is indicated for all those with a definite history of anaphylaxis and in children with asthma on inhaled steroids who have less severe reactions because they are at greater risk of anaphylaxis. Routine prescription for all children with a history of a peanut or nut allergy is controversial. Mild reactions to foodstuffs are very common and avoidance is the key.

 KEY POINT

- Intramuscular adrenaline is the first-line treatment for acute anaphylaxis.

CASE 97: A PREGNANT 14-YEAR-OLD

History

Anna is a 14-year-old girl who presents to her GP worried that she may be pregnant. She started her periods at the age of 11 and they have been pretty regular, but she has now missed two and has been suffering from nausea most mornings. She met a 19-year-old man called Ryan at a party 6 months ago and they have been seeing each other since, mainly at his flat which he shares with three other people, but occasionally at her house when her parents are at work. She remembers a night a couple of months ago when she and Ryan had had a few drinks and the condom slipped off. They thought it would be fine. He works as a chef and she has been playing truant and missing school if he is working in the evening. Up until now she has been doing well at school, but she anticipates that her grades will slip this year.

Ryan is not her first sexual partner and she has always relied on condoms as she is worried that the contraceptive pill will make her put on weight. Anna has not told her family about Ryan knowing that they will disapprove. She has no significant past medical history. Unfortunately, Ryan is also a smoker and she has started smoking cigarettes. She denies taking any other recreational drugs. Anna is adamant that she does not want the baby and is equally adamant that she does not want to involve her parents or Ryan in any decision about a termination. None of them knows she is seeing the GP.

Examination

Anna is generally healthy. There is nothing abnormal to find on examination and the uterus is not palpable.

INVESTIGATIONS
Urine β-human chorionic gonadotrophin is positive.

Questions
- Where does the GP stand legally regarding Anna and Ryan's relationship?
- May Anna make up her own mind about a termination?

ANSWER 97

Ryan has broken the Sexual Offences Act (2003) by having sexual intercourse with a young person under 16 years. However, the Act aims to reduce sexual exploitation and abuse of children and young people, not to criminalize normal adolescent behaviour. If all young people known to be sexually active were reported to the police, they would probably be less likely to access contraceptive and sexual health services, leaving them more vulnerable to unintended pregnancy and other health risks. Under the Act, all those under 16 have the right to confidential advice, and the person offering it, medical or non-medical, is not guilty of any offence, provided they are protecting the child's physical and/or emotional well-being.

The key words are 'exploitation' and 'abuse', and in the rare event of these being present, the patient must understand that absolute confidentiality cannot be guaranteed. To determine whether a relationship presents a risk that needs referral to Social Care and/or police, the GP needs to consider:

- whether the young person is competent to understand and consent to the sexual activity – according to the Act, children under 13 are not and anyone involved in penetrative sex can be convicted of rape
- power imbalances through differences in size, age and development – even 16 and 17-year-olds cannot give informed consent if the perpetrator is in a position of trust, such as a teacher or youth worker
- whether there was aggression, manipulation or bribery including the use of drugs and/or alcohol
- attempts to secure unreasonable secrecy
- whether the partner is known by agencies to have worrying relationships with other young people
- evidence of parental neglect or lack of supervision in a child under 13
- whether the relationship involves behaviours considered to be 'grooming' in the context of sexual exploitation.

From Anna's history there are no obvious legal or safeguarding children's anxieties about her relationship with Ryan, although it is far from ideal. Therefore the GP does not have to report it to anyone.

In UK law the legal age of consent to medical treatment is 16 years. There is a legal precedent for younger children to give valid consent provided they fulfil approved criteria. To be 'Gillick' competent they must demonstrate sufficient maturity and intelligence (capacity) to understand the nature and implications of the proposed treatment, including the risks and alternatives, and the consequences of not having it.

This means that Anna could have a termination without her parents' (or her boyfriend's) knowledge, although she should be actively encouraged to tell them.

Note that a child is not considered to have the capacity to refuse investigation or treatment against the judgment of their parents or doctors. A 15-year-old cannot refuse blood tests or treatment, although every effort should be made to understand their fears and wishes.

KEY POINTS

- All children under 16 years have the right to confidential sexual health advice.
- Only where there is evidence of exploitation or abuse should cases of underage sex be referred to Social Care and/or police.
- Young people can, under specific circumstances, consent to treatment independently of their parents but they should always be encouraged to involve them.

History

Zara is a 4-month-old infant who is brought to the A&E department and taken straight to the resuscitation bay. Her parents say that they had gone to bed with Zara lying in the bed between them and when they woke up she was blue, not breathing and lifeless. She had been generally well the previous day but had not fed as well as usual. Zara was born at 32 weeks gestation, weighing 1.90 kg, and had been in the special care baby unit for 5 weeks. She had required oxygen for 2 days and had been nasogastrically fed for 3 weeks. The parents are not consanguineous and Zara is their first child.

The ambulance crew state that the baby was not breathing and asystolic when they arrived. Zara has had basic life support during the 10-min journey to the hospital.

Examination

There is no respiratory rate and no air entry. Oxygen saturation is unrecordable. There is no heart rate and a flat ECG trace. The baby is limp and unresponsive, with a temperature of 35.8°C.

Questions
- What is your immediate management?
- Which investigations should be performed?
- What is the likely outcome?
- How would you proceed if the child did not survive?

ANSWER 98

Basic life support with CPR should be continued and the Advanced Paediatric Life Support asystole algorithm should be followed (see Fig. 98.1).

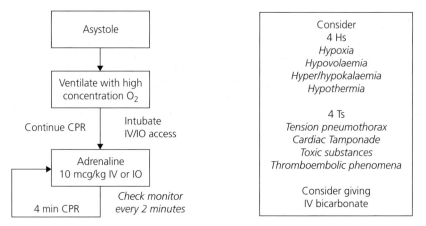

Figure 98.1 Advanced Paediatric Life Support asystole algorithm. (Reproduced with modifications from APLS manual, with permission from ALSG and Blackwell Publishing.)

Investigations need to be wide ranging, looking into possibilities such as sepsis, metabolic disease and poisoning. A bedside glucose measurement should be done immediately. It is not always possible to get sufficient blood and urine for all the tests:

- *Blood tests*: full blood count, urea and electrolytes, bone chemistry, liver function tests, glucose, C-reactive protein, blood gas, blood culture, ammonia, lactate, amino acids, toxicology, cross-match
- *Urine tests*: microscopy, culture and sensitivity, amino acids, organic acids, toxicology
- *Nasopharyngeal aspirate* for virology and bacteriology.
- *Chest X-ray* and any other imaging as indicated.

The likely outcome is death. Cardiac arrest in children is rarely due to cardiac disease and is usually secondary to hypoxia ± acidosis due to a respiratory illness, e.g. bronchiolitis.

Schindler *et al.* (N Engl J Med 1996; 335: 1473–9) published data on the outcome of out-of-hospital cardiorespiratory arrests. It showed that the absence of any response after 20 min of full hospital resuscitation resulted in 100 per cent mortality. It is conventional to resuscitate infants in hospital for 30 min. An overly prolonged resuscitation can result in the survival of an infant with very severe neurological damage. Rarely, following drowning or poisoning, resuscitation for longer than 30 min is necessary.

If the child does not survive, the parents need to be talked to sensitively and told that all sudden unexpected deaths in infancy (SUDI, the new name for the sudden infant death syndrome which was previously also known as cot death) are referred to the coroner and that the baby by law requires a postmortem. The parents also need to be told that it is possible that no cause will be found for the death. They should be told that the police will be automatically informed. The child protection register should be checked. Most hospitals have a list of people who need to be informed after an infant has died, e.g. general practitioner.

The family need to be followed up to discuss the results of the postmortem. Bereavement counselling should also be offered.

KEY POINTS
• Cardiac arrest in children is usually secondary to hypoxia due to respiratory disease.
• Following an out-of-hospital cardiac arrest, lack of a response after 20 min of hospital resuscitation almost invariably results in death.
• All cases of SUDI require a referral to the coroner and a postmortem.

History

Charlotte is 14 years old. She is referred to the paediatric outpatient department by her GP. Over the last 6 months she has been complaining of feeling tired all the time, she has a sore throat, headaches, pains in her arms, legs and abdomen, and feels weak. She has not been to school for the last 6 weeks because she can't manage the walk to the bus stop and now she needs her mother's assistance to walk around her house. The referral letter says that they have attended the GP's surgery five times over this period, and the mother is very anxious about what is causing this. The GP did some blood tests and says that a full blood count, renal and liver function tests were normal.

Further history reveals that this all started with a sore throat and fever for a few days. From then on, she started to get headaches, worse in the evening, and became weak and lethargic. She seemed to get worse each week, until she was hardly doing anything herself, staying in bed or watching television. Despite sleeping a lot, she doesn't feel refreshed after sleeping. Her mother has to help her to shower and dress, as she feels so weak. She aches all over and finds it very hard to concentrate on anything. Her periods have become irregular.

Charlotte was getting top grades at school before all this and wants to be a doctor. She enjoys school and denies any bullying. She lives with her mother and stepfather. She has always been very reliant on her mother. Her sister was successfully treated for acute lymphoblastic leukaemia 3 years ago. Charlotte has never been in hospital before and usually does swimming team training five times per week.

Her mother is very worried that this could be something sinister and she has looked on the internet and thinks it could be a brain tumour or thyroid problem. She is upset that the GP hasn't taken it seriously and only did blood tests because she made a fuss.

Examination

Charlotte is rather quiet, but will participate in conversation when prompted. Her weight is 45 kg (25th centile) and her height is 164 cm (75th centile). Otherwise, physical examination is unremarkable.

Questions
- What is the most likely diagnosis?
- Would you request any more investigations?
- What is the prognosis?

ANSWER 99

The most likely diagnosis is chronic fatigue syndrome (CFS). This condition is also known as myalgic encephalopathy (ME), but the term CFS is now preferred. The cause of this condition is unknown. The diagnosis requires persistent fatigue disrupting daily life for 6 months, associated with typical symptoms and no underlying cause found by routine investigation. Typical symptoms include malaise, headache, nausea, sore throat, painful lymph nodes, myalgia, abdominal pain, poor sleep and poor concentration. Teenagers are more often affected than younger children.

This girl's personality, social and emotional background are probably predisposing factors. It is necessary to exclude organic pathology early on, and to demonstrate that the symptoms are being taken seriously. At the same time it is important to indicate from the start that CFS could be the cause of all these symptoms. Thorough physical examination should include lying and standing heart rates and blood pressure, neurological assessment and examination for lymphadenopathy, hepatosplenomegaly, tonsil abnormalities and sinusitis. Investigations should rule out active infection, inflammation, endocrine problems and malignancy. When headache is prominent, it may be necessary to perform an MRI scan of the brain to exclude a space-occupying lesion.

!	Recommended investigations in patients suspected to have CFS	
		May indicate:
	Full blood count and blood film	Anaemia/leukaemia
	Erythrocyte sedimentation rate and C-reactive protein	Inflammatory/infectious cause
	Urea, creatinine	Renal disease
	Glucose and electrolytes	Endocrine disease, e.g. Addison's
	Creatine kinase	Myositis
	Liver function	Hepatitis
	Thyroid function	Hypothyroidism
	Urine dipstick	Diabetes mellitus, renal disease
	Epstein–Barr Virus (EBV) serology	Current EBV infection

Prognosis is quite variable and although two-thirds of patients make a full recovery, this may take 3–4 years. A multidisciplinary approach is often required. Management begins with assessment of baseline function using an activity diary. Supportive treatment can be aimed at alleviating symptoms, improving nutrition and sleep patterns and preventing over-exertion. A graded programme of return to activity is often instituted once a stable baseline has been achieved. Support from physiotherapy, occupational therapy and child and adolescent mental health services may also be needed. Occasionally in-patient management is required for investigation, evaluation and planning of treatment.

In this case, Charlotte was admitted to the paediatric ward for about 4 weeks, initially for investigation, and then for some intensive assessment by physiotherapists, occupational therapists and child and adolescent mental health services. It was difficult to make Charlotte and her mother accept the diagnosis of CFS. She was discharged after her baseline activity level had been established and a programme of rehabilitation had been planned. She had regular follow-up to support her in achieving her goals. After

18 months she has returned to about 60 per cent of her previous activity levels, and continues to make slow progress. She has dropped back 1 year at school, but now manages to attend most of her lessons.

🔑 | **KEY POINTS**

- Chronic fatigue syndrome can be a debilitating condition requiring a multidisciplinary approach.
- Chronic fatigue and associated features should have been present for at least 6 months.
- Other medical causes of the same symptoms should be excluded.

History

Charlie is a 14-month-old boy who is referred by his GP to the paediatric day unit because of diarrhoea and weight loss. He has had numerous previous admissions. Charlie was born at 32 weeks after a pregnancy complicated by recurrent bleeding. He needed headbox oxygen for 5 days. By discharge home at 6 weeks, he was bottle-fed and his weight was on the 25th centile. Over the next 2 months he had several admissions with possible apnoeas, but investigations including an EEG and brain MRI were normal and none were witnessed during observation on the ward. At 4 months he had two episodes of haematemesis confirmed on inspection of the towels his mother brought with her and had a normal full blood count, clotting screen and barium meal. His weight by then had dropped to the 2nd centile and it has not been above it since, and has occasionally fallen to below the 0.4th centile.

He has persistent, frequent, loose stools often containing visible blood. A diagnosis of cow's milk protein intolerance was made, but a dairy-free diet made no difference. He is now on a hydrolysated (pre-digested) formula. Solids were introduced at 5 months.

During his admissions the nurses have fed him and report that he is always hungry and takes good amounts, but there has been no significant weight gain. Charlie has had extensive normal investigations, including an abdominal ultrasound, small bowel biopsy and a colonoscopy, when no blood was seen. There are no concerns about his development. His 4-year-old brother was also investigated for poor weight gain. With the permission of the parents, reports have been obtained from the tertiary centre to which the 4-year-old was referred – he, too, had exhaustive tests but no diagnosis was ever made. His growth chart shows a rapid improvement in weight gain from about 2 years. Charlie's mother is a pharmacy technician and his father is a lorry driver. The staff know them well and his mother is always happy to stay.

Examination

Charlie looks skinny. He has redundant skin folds over his thighs and buttocks. His weight is just below the 0.4th centile, and his length and head circumference are on the 50th centiles. He is not clubbed and not clinically anaemic. His pulse is 180 beats/min. Examination is otherwise unremarkable.

Questions

- What is the most likely diagnosis?
- What could be the mechanisms contributing to Charlie's history and current clinical state?
- What should happen next?

ANSWER 100

Charlie has had several unexplained episodes of potentially serious illness and now has evidence of ongoing faltering weight gain with blood in his stools but not at colonoscopy. Exhaustive investigations are normal. This is on the background of being born preterm after a complicated pregnancy and having an older brother who had a similar pattern of illness in the first 2 years of life. This is all highly consistent with a diagnosis of fabricated or induced illness (FII), an uncommon and difficult to diagnose form of child abuse. The perpetrator may:

- fabricate a medical history
- cause symptoms by repeatedly exposing the child to a toxin, medication, infectious agent or physical trauma, including smothering
- alter laboratory samples or temperature measurements.

The mother is almost always responsible and a significant percentage have connections with the health services. Sadly the disturbed parent seems to obtain a perverse satisfaction from the close association with hospital care and staff. The possible mechanisms in this case include the blood in the vomit and stools being his mother's, possibly even her menstrual blood. Specimens can be analysed for 'foreign' blood. The vaginal bleeding during pregnancy may have been self-induced. The apnoeas could have many explanations and covert surveillance by the police may be needed if episodes are ongoing and smothering is a possibility. Faltering weight gain means that energy expenditure exceeds energy intake. Possibilities include diluting his feeds, throwing feeds away or poisoning with laxatives or an agent that increases metabolic rate such as thyroxine – to which this mother, as a pharmacy technician, would have access. This possibility is supported by his tachycardia. Thyrotoxicosis is extraordinarily rare in this age group and thyroid function tests may be normal if doses are not given every day. Some mothers become highly sophisticated at FII – and this mother may have had prior experience with her older boy. A phone call to the GP may reveal a history of abuse during the mother's childhood or prior mental health problems, but these do not mean that this is FII. It is all supportive, not diagnostic, evidence.

However, it is crucial to make the diagnosis because this disorder can be very damaging to the child, not just from the impact of the unnecessary and invasive investigations but because of long-term behavioural and other problems. Other children may also be at risk. The case must be referred to Social Care, who have a statutory duty to undertake a thorough investigation according to strict guidelines. The child protection register should be checked and the health visitor should be contacted for further information. At the same time, it is worth obtaining a second opinion from another consultant paediatrician.

 KEY POINTS

- Fabricated and induced illness should be considered in any child with recurrent unexplained symptoms, but it may be difficult to diagnose.
- All potential cases of fabricated and induced illness must be referred to Social Care.

INDEX

References are by case number with relevant page number(s) following in brackets. References with a page range e.g. 25(68–70) indicate that although the subject may be mentioned only on one page, it concerns the whole case.